PROMOTING WELLNESS

Beyond Hormone Therapy

Options For Prostate Cancer Patients

Mark A. Moyad, MD, MPH

This book is dedicated to my dad and doctor, Robert Moyad. He taught me what it means to put patients first and what it means to be a good husband and father.

It is also dedicated to the individuals—Epstein, Jenkins, Pokempner, and Thompson—who invest in the dream and allow me to make a difference one starfish at a time.

Another group that deserves credit are all of the oncologists, urologists, and other health care professionals from around the world whom I consulted with during the preparation of this book. I cannot thank you enough for your passion and dedication to your patients, your overall guidance, your objective critiques of the manuscript, and your friendship.

And finally, this book is dedicated to the advocates, advocacy groups, health care professionals, patients, and their families who have battled and are still fighting prostate cancer.

All inquiries should be addressed to:
Spry Publishing, an imprint of Ann Arbor Editions, LLC,
2500 S. State Street,
Ann Arbor, MI 48104

www.annarboreditions.com
877-722-2264

Printed in the United States of America

ISBN: 978-1-58726-682-9

---

10 9 8 7 6 5 4 3 2 1

CONTENTS

Introduction

LET KNOWLEDGE EMPOWER YOU

WELCOME to a unique educational book for individuals dealing with advanced prostate cancer, those with a rising PSA after being on hormone or androgen deprivation therapy (ADT). This book is intended to complement *Promoting Wellness for Prostate Cancer Patients*, which is currently available and has been circulated around the world for almost a decade. Hormone refractory prostate cancer (HRPC), or as we're calling it "Beyond Hormonal Therapy," is a stage of the disease that currently has so many options that it needed its own separate book. Most prostate cancer resources focus on the needs of individuals with localized prostate cancer, leaving a void of information for those men needing further treatment. Our primary goal with this book is to empower you with information and suggestions to assist you in communicating with your doctor and other health-care professionals while dealing with your cancer. Through that informed communication, you and your physician will select the treatment options that best suit your individual needs.

Section one is a quick review. We start chapter one with questions commonly asked by advanced prostate cancer patients. We'll discuss how the cancer came to be advanced, what factors affect prognosis, and, generally speaking, what treatments are available. Chapters two and three will cover secondary hormonal treatments and other therapies that are used either before or in addition to the U.S. Food and Drug Administration–approved (FDA-approved) treatments in the section that follows. In chapters four through eight, we will present current cutting-edge treatment information that will allow you to control and hopefully beat this disease. For the upcoming therapies in chapter eight, we've focused on those coming in the near future, several months away as opposed to several years away.

Use this book to help you develop questions and understand state-of-the-art treatments. We want this book to give you and the individuals who love and support you the extra knowledge to hit this disease with anything and everything out there. Always remember, in dealing with your health, knowledge and action equals power!

Chapter nine will help you anticipate and mitigate the potential side effects of the various treatments. Understanding and alleviating those effects will improve your comfort during treatment. We'll consider lifestyle changes, nutritional options, supplements, and prescription medications to give you a variety of choices.

In chapter ten, we'll review diet, supplements, and alternative medicinal therapies that can enhance your well-being, both during treatment and in general. Finally, we'll give you a quick overview of some of the drugs potentially coming in the more distant future, along with some treatments approved for another disease that may be helpful in advanced prostate cancer as well.

As you reach the end of the book, hopefully you'll have a new wealth of knowledge to consider and discuss with your health-care providers in setting up the best care plan for your situation. This is the most optimistic time for men with hormone-refractory prostate cancer, with new treatments testing all the time. Just remember, especially in dealing with cancer, combining knowledge and action really equals power!

Mark A. Moyad, MD, MPH
Jenkins/Pokempner Director of
Preventive & Alternative Medicine
University of Michigan Medical Center–
Department of Urology

Consulting Director of Medical Education & Research
Eisenhower Wellness Institute

A Quick *and* Necessary Review

Questions *and* Answers *to* Start

Chapter One

When a patient is confronted with prostate cancer that is advancing, certain important questions come to mind almost immediately. It seemed to make the most sense to put those questions on the table first and provide some general answers before we get into more depth in upcoming chapters.

Question 1: What is hormone-refractory prostate cancer (HRPC)?

Men most commonly are considered to have hormone-refractory prostate cancer when their prostate specific antigen level, or PSA, starts to rise while on hormone therapy (also called androgen deprivation therapy [ADT] or luteinizing hormone-releasing hormone therapy [LHRH]). However, a small number of men are diagnosed with an advanced stage of prostate cancer prior to receiving any treatment. They are offered ADT the moment the physician finds prostate cancer well beyond the prostate—for example, in the bones.

Over the years, several names have been given to the advanced cancer condition involving a rising PSA after hormone therapy, but in reality all of the names represent somewhat similar stages of prostate cancer. You may hear any of the terms below used:

Androgen-Independent Prostate Cancer (AIPC) The cancer no longer depends on the androgen receptor or androgen signaling for growth and survival.

Castrate-Resistant Prostate Cancer (CRPC) The cancer continues to grow and progress even though a man has only castrate levels of testosterone or male hormone (less than 50 ng/dL [1.7 nmol/L]).

Hormone-Refractory Prostate Cancer (HRPC) The cancer no longer responds to hormone therapy (LHRH, for example). For simplicity, we will use HRPC throughout this book.

Question 2: How did my cancer become "hormone-refractory"?

Unfortunately, despite hormone therapy, some prostate cancers continue to progress, and more treatment is needed. Those treatments might include options such as second- and third-line hormone therapies, chemotherapy, or, perhaps, even an immune therapy recently approved by the FDA.

So what actually happens when prostate cancer that responded to ADT turns into HRPC? Why does this occur? Several things can bring about this change:

- There may be increases in the expression of a gene that can keep the tumor alive (known as up-regulation of survival genes), or an increase in the amount (amplification) or the appearance of different types (mutations) of the androgen receptors expressed by the tumor. As a result, the tumor can survive on less testosterone.
- Other unique compounds are activated, accepted, or even produced by the tumor to keep the cancer alive.
- The tumor acquires the ability to create its own concentration of testosterone, bypassing the ADT treatment.
- The cancer alters the body's control panels and acquires the ability to "feed" itself, so to speak, by creating a blood supply directly into the tumor (a process called angiogenesis). In this process, the tumor may become resistant to specific drugs or even use these drugs as its own fuel.
- The cancer becomes able to evade the body's immune system and the body no longer recognizes that it has a tumor growing. The tumor can do this by causing changes that keep the immune cells in an immature state, allowing the tumor to move throughout the body without detection.

HRPC patients wage a battle against regular adaptations to the tumor that may occur during the course of treatment.

The tumor's ability to use all or some of these adaptations is what has made it challenging to develop effective treatments for this stage of the disease. Researchers are always working to stay one step ahead of this sequence of events. In the following chapters, we'll focus much more on treatment options. However, the good news is that more effective treatment options are available now.

Question 3: Should I continue ADT or hormone deprivation treatment going forward?

ADT or hormone therapy works by shutting off most of the testosterone production in the testicles, either through the use of drug treatments or by surgically removing the testicles. Since testosterone has a role in tumor growth, removing testosterone can slow or stop the tumor growth in many cases. Let's consider for a moment how that process works.

Most prostate cancers have an androgen receptor (AR), a place where testosterone is accepted or recognized by the tumor so that it can grow. One primary way to contain the tumor is by simply removing the testosterone that can fit the AR. It is well established that the growth and survival of prostate tumors, at least for a certain period of time, is dependent on the continued stimulation of the androgen receptor by testosterone. This is why ADT, which eliminates testosterone, has been one of the most successful treatments for more than twenty years.

The initial goal with ADT is to reach *castrate levels of testosterone*, or less than 50 ng/dL (1.7 nmol/L). However, some experts believe the desired level should be less than 20 ng/dL (0.7 nmol/L). ADT is one of the primary treatments against metastatic prostate cancer and is used along with radiation for more aggressive (high-risk) or locally advanced prostate cancer (cancer that has gone beyond the prostate). Unfortunately, when patients have metastatic disease, the primary response to ADT alone can be temporary. Some men respond for years and years, and others respond for a shorter time.

When patients ask about remaining on ADT after the primary response fails, it is worth pointing out that remaining on hormone therapy can increase the chances of living longer. A study has shown an increased and significant survival advantage for men who did remain on hormone therapy despite having a rising PSA. Also, most clinical trials of new drug treatments require patients to stay on hormone therapy if they want to participate in the trial. Lastly, many leading cancer doctors believe that hormone therapy, despite a rising PSA, continues to provide benefits such as immunity-boosting and the continuous killing of hormone-sensitive cells. In summary, it is worth considering three points:

- Research has shown that, even if the PSA is rising, there are still cancer cells that may respond to testosterone produced by the body. ADT can help kill those cells on a regular basis.
- Research also shows that there may be a slight reduction in symptoms and a greater survival benefit if a man stays on ADT.
- Most clinical trials require men to stay on ADT to enroll, so remaining on hormone therapy keeps options open for your treatment.

Question 4: What is my prognosis right now?

Certainly, one of the most common questions after being diagnosed with HRPC relates to how long you can be expected to live with the disease. The answer is that no one really knows for sure. We do know, however, that this is the most optimistic research period for HRPC in history. Just since the writing of this book began, the U.S. Food and Drug Administration has approved 3 new drugs for HRPC, and two have the potential of extending patients' lives.

Some individuals call advanced prostate cancer "stage 4" cancer. This is both inaccurate and misleading for it implies that there is a lack of options and that your quality and quantity of life will be very poor. *In fact, most men at this stage of the disease can still respond very well to a whole range of options currently available, such as secondary hormonal therapies, immune therapy, chemotherapy, or a clinical trial of a promising therapy.*

The various factors listed below all play roles in determining how well someone with HRPC will do. Some men have very aggressive HRPC, while other cancers are not as aggressive. Some patients respond very well to treatment, and others do not respond so well. Generally, the following factors are considered in determining a treatment course for a patient. Bear in mind that no single factor is a clear indicator of success or failure. Just because one or more of the factors below may be associated with a worse prognosis does not indicate a shorter life span, but it may mean that discussions with your doctor will involve different options appropriate for your individual situation. In other words, knowing that your cancer may be more aggressive can give you a better indication of how aggressively you want to have your cancer treated.

Prognostic Indicators To Discusss With Your Doctor

Age Age has very little impact by itself on whether or not you would qualify for or respond to a HRPC treatment. Overall, older men tend to respond just as well as younger men to HRPC treatment. However, younger men diagnosed with HRPC tend to have a worse prognosis simply because they have more aggressive tumors in some cases. And, since they are expected to have a longer life span, and since fewer currently have other health issues, HRPC does have a greater chance of eventually impacting them. In other words, older men are more likely to also have other serious diseases (co-morbidities, such as heart disease, diabetes, and other cancers) that could affect their lifes during the time they are being treated for HRPC.

Albumin This is an important protein in the blood that is measured by a blood test. It serves as a carrier for all sorts of vital substances in the human body. A normal albumin level is a good indicator that the body is doing well when receiving treatment, but an abnormally low albumin level could be an indicator that the patient is not doing as well.

Alkaline Phosphatase A blood test for alkaline phosphatase measures the quantity of an important enzyme in the body that can help to predict the aggressiveness of your HRPC, as well as what the cancer is doing to your body. An abnormally high level of this enzyme tends to suggest that the cancer is being more aggressive and is not responding as well to treatment.

Asymptomatic or Symptomatic There are two distinctly different clinical stages within HRPC, namely, individuals who are **ASYMPTOMATIC** (experiencing no symptoms at all) and **SYMPTOMATIC** (experiencing some symptoms). Thanks to the PSA test and better imaging tests, the majority of men currently diagnosed with HRPC are asymptomatic. This is because the disease is being detected earlier and earlier, opening up more treatment options for HRPC patients. Men with asymptomatic HRPC have a better prognosis, in general. However, this may change somewhat in the future as more and more drug treatment options for men with symptomatic HRPC are in clinical trials right now.

Bone Metastasis and Number of Bone Metastases In general, individuals with HRPC who have bone metastasis (cancer that has spread to the bone) have a cancer that has progressed further than that of someone with no bone metastasis. Individuals with more bone metastasis could have a worse prognosis or a more serious HRPC, for the cancer has spread to more places in the body. In addition, when cancer spreads to unusual bone sites, such as the skull, new data suggest that such spread is associated with a more aggressive cancer.

Bone-Protecting Medication There is some preliminary indication in other types of advanced cancer that receiving a bone drug to reduce the risk of bone loss after being diagnosed may also reduce the risk of bone metastasis and improve survival. Studies are preliminary, but it appears that protecting your bones after being diagnosed with HRPC is critical to reducing the risk of bone loss that could delay your cancer treatment.

Circulating Tumor Cells The practice of monitoring circulating tumor cells (CTCs) to assess the effectiveness of a treatment or give some indication of prognosis is starting to get some attention. CTCs are epithelial cells that actually come free or are shed from different tumors. These CTCs can be counted in a new blood test (for example, "cell search"; see www.veridex.com). This test is being used in some clinical trials right now, and there seems to be an indication that when a drug causes a reduction in CTCs during treatment, or when there are fewer CTCs before the treatment, there is an increase in survival rates. This makes sense, because a reduction in tumor cells probably means that some cells have been destroyed. Ask your doctor about this new test if you are interested.

Diet, Lifestyle Changes, and Over-The-Counter Medicines Whether or not any diet or supplements could improve your HRPC prognosis specifically has not been proven, but a man who exercises regularly, eats a moderately healthy diet, and maintains a healthy weight may reduce his risk of getting other diseases that can reduce his life expectancy. A recent study of men diagnosed with HRPC found that a large number of men actually die yearly from other causes, such as cardiovascular disease. In the diet and supplement section of the book, you will find heart-healthy tips that may fight prostate cancer and a list of dietary supplements to consider taking or to avoid based on research on their likely effect on prognosis.

Gleason Total Score and Primary Gleason Score A higher total Gleason score (scores of 8 to 10, for example) indicates a more aggressive cancer. Prognosis or response to a drug could be worse for someone with this type of tumor as compared with someone who has a moderate or low Gleason score (below 8, for example). Most Gleason scores on tumors were established a long time ago for men with more localized disease, but knowing this number is still helpful in making treatment decisions. Some researchers believe that the first number in your Gleason score, called the primary Gleason score, is as important as the total Gleason score. For example, a primary Gleason score of 4 or 5 suggests a worse prognosis as compared to a primary score of 3. A man with a Gleason total score of 5 + 3 = 8 may have a worse prognosis as compared to someone with a score of 4 + 4 = 8.

Hemoglobin A hemoglobin count is a measure of the oxygen-carrying protein in your red blood cells. If hemoglobin is very low (a situation called anemia), a person may feel tired, and it will be more difficult for him to receive treatment. It is not unusual to be slightly anemic due to testosterone-lowering treatments, but an abnormally low hemoglobin level that causes a variety of symptoms (fatigue, breathing problems, etc.) may need to be treated. It can make the prognosis slightly worse by causing a delay in cancer treatments.

Hormone Treatment (LHRH, ADT, or Surgical Castration) As we discussed earlier, maintaining a castrate level of testosterone is recommended for most HRPC patients. This may provide both quality- and quantity-of-life benefits. But is it better to reduce testosterone by using regular LHRH injections, or just to have the testicles surgically removed? There has been no strong research to show that there is a survival or prognostic advantage of one method over the other. However, in some surveys of patients there seems to be a quality-of-life benefit for those who receive regular LHRH injections. Patients visit their doctors frequently to receive the injection, and that may be a positive thing. The injection may provide the patient with a feeling of control over the process and allow him to avoid surgery to permanently remove the testicles. It is worth noting that most patients who take LHRH injections for a period of time will not start to produce testosterone again, even if the injections are stopped. A patient who has to travel long distances to receive the injections may benefit from surgery.

Imaging Test Results X-rays, bone scans, CT scans, MRIs, or any other imaging tests that show that the cancer is spreading to more body sites tend to indicate that the cancer is more aggressive and not responding to treatment. Cancer that is not spreading or tumors that are shrinking in size are both good indicators that the patient is responding to treatment. (More information on imaging tests can be found in the appendices at the end of the book.)

Lactate Dehydrogenase Also known as LDH, this is an important enzyme in the body that can be measured in a blood test and can help to predict the aggressiveness of your HRPC or what the cancer will do to your body. An abnormally high level of this enzyme tends to suggest that the cancer is more aggressive and is not responding as well to treatment.

Medical History and Co-morbidities It makes sense that your general health and any other diagnosed diseases (co-morbidities) can have an impact on your prognosis. Not surprisingly, individuals with other serious disease besides prostate cancer have a greater chance of dying younger. Individuals who are healthier in general and who have few to no co-morbidities tend to live longer. For example, obesity does not seem to impact HRPC prognosis, but it does increase the risk of dying younger from other causes, such as cardiovascular disease. Keeping other disease states under control, as much as possible, and maintaining general health through exercise and proper diet makes a lot of sense.

Pain Men with HRPC and different pain levels tend to have different prognoses. The worse the pain caused by the cancer itself, the worse the prognosis or the more serious the situation. This makes sense because tumors that have grown large enough to cause pain are more troubling than smaller tumors not causing pain. Pain caused by other chronic conditions, such as arthritis, does not play a role in this consideration.

Performance Status Performance status is a scale that attempts to quantify the general well-being or quality of life of a patient. Health-care professionals use the scale to determine whether someone should receive chemotherapy treatment, whether a dosage change is needed, or if therapy should even be continued for a particular patient. Two commonly used scales are the ECOG (Eastern Cooperative Oncology Group, one of the largest clinical cancer research organizations in the United States) test and the Karnofsky Performance Status test (named for Dr. David A. Karnofsky). A brief description of each follows. Overall, a poor performance status indicates a worse prognosis as compared to someone with a better performance status.

ECOG Performance Status

Numerous clinical trials require an ECOG performance status of 0 to 2 in order to be allowed to participate in clinical trials. Scores of 3 or 4 usually do not receive chemotherapy because the possibility of benefit is outweighed by the potential of negative side effects (of course, there are exceptions).

0 Asymptomatic (fully active, no restrictions)

1 Symptomatic and fully able to walk (can perform light work, such as household or office tasks, but cannot do strenuous activity)

2 Symptomatic and spends less than 50 percent of time in bed (can walk and provide self-care, but unable to do work activities)

3 Symptomatic and spends more than 50 percent of time

in bed or chair (not bedbound, capable of limited self-care)

4 Bedbound (cannot provide for self-care, completely confined to bed or chair)

Karnofsky Performance Status

Can be expressed as a range (90–100) or a specific number (92).

- 100 Normal, no complaints or signs of disease
- 90 Normal activity, few symptoms or signs of disease
- 80 Normal activity, some symptoms or signs of disease
- 70 Caring for self, not capable of normal activity or work
- 60 Needs some help, can take care of personal requirements
- 50 Needs help often, requires frequent medical care
- 40 Disabled, needs special help and care
- 30 Severely disabled, hospital admission indicated but no danger of death
- 20 Very ill, urgently needing admission, needs supportive measures of treatment
- 10 Rapidly progressive

Previous Response To Treatment(s) Response to previous HRPC treatments is a good indicator of prognosis or the aggressiveness of your tumor. For example, someone who responded well to several cycles of Taxotere chemotherapy has a better prognosis as compared to someone who responded for a short time or not at all. A patient who had a positive PSA response to several anti-androgens or secondary hormonal therapies has a better prognosis in general than someone who did not respond to any of them. Positive response to one drug treatment for HRPC is a good indicator that this same individual could respond favorably to other treatments.

Primary Tumor Site Status or Debulking This is a very controversial prognostic indicator. A number of opinions exist, and there are no clear answers as of this time, but it is a topic you may want to discuss with your doctor. In some other tumor types, such as colon and ovarian, a person with advanced cancer may have a better prognosis when the primary tumor or the location where the tumor initially began to grow is removed (debulked). It appears that removing the ovaries or part of the colon even though a patient has cancer that has spread far beyond these areas could still provide a benefit. How? Simply removing part of the primary tumor may make it less able to send out more cancer cells into the rest of the body or even communicate with other tumor cells in the body. Does this mean that men with HRPC should get their prostate removed or get radiation to the prostate again? While there is no definitive answer at this time, it may be worth discussing with your doctor.

Prostatic Acid Phosphatase (PAP) Historically, this blood test was used before the PSA test was invented to determine whether someone had prostate cancer. However, the prostatic acid phosphatase (PAP) number only increased to large values when the disease had already spread to different areas of the body, making early detection difficult. Some doctors still use this test once in a while to determine if HRPC is more extensive when they cannot find any tumors on the imaging devices. While this test may complement the prognostic value of the PSA in some rare situations, it does not tell the doctor more than what the other tests are showing for most patients.

PSA and PSA Kinetics Increasing PSA, rapidly increasing PSA, or a PSA that does not respond to a treatment could all be indicators of a worse prognosis, but keep in mind that there are exceptions to this rule. For example, Provenge treatment for HRPC does not necessarily reduce PSA levels, but it is associated with a greater survival rate. On the other hand, Taxotere chemotherapy tends to lower PSA or slow the rise in PSA in many men, and it is also associated with an improved survival for HRPC. There are also cases where very aggressive tumors don't produce PSA, and where less aggressive tumors create a higher PSA. Considering both your PSA before treatment and location of the tumor in the body may provide some guidance.

PSA kinetics (doubling time, velocity) may also be useful. For example, the longer it takes for PSA to double after treatment, the more likely it is to be a favorable prognostic sign.

Race and Ethnicity may have an impact on prognosis for many reasons. Past studies have indicated that non-Caucasian men or minorities tend to have less access to health care or are more likely to have their treatment delayed. Improved education and health care access may resolve this factor in the future.

Staging of Cancer Staging is a system used to identify where a cancer is located and how far it has spread. The TNM staging system is the most common one used for prostate cancer. The acronym stands for primary tumor location (T), lymph nodes (N), and metastases (M). The tumor location is based on the results of a clinical examination, imaging tests, a biopsy, and blood tests. The node assessment is generally based on a clinical examination, imaging, or lymph node removal. The assessment of metastases utilizes clinical examination, imaging, specific bone or skeletal studies, and blood tests. Every prostate cancer should be given a T, N, and M assessment. An "x" or "0" score for the T, N, or M indicator usually means that either the location of the tumor cannot be determined currently (for example, Tx, Nx, or Mx), or there is no evidence of cancer in that area after evaluation (for example, T0, N0, or M0). Subcategories can be used to provide a more exact tumor location, but those subcategories won't be covered here because in treating hormone-refractory cancer patients more emphasis is placed on the N and M staging. Not surprisingly, patients with a higher TNM stage have a worse prognosis than patients with a low TNM stage.

Primary Tumor Location (T stage)	What does this mean?
T1	Tumor is within the prostate and found only by PSA and biopsy alone, or using another non-cancer prostate procedure (for example TURP), but was not found by imaging or digital rectal exam.
T2	Tumor is within the prostate and found by digital rectal exam, combined digital rectal exam and PSA testing, imaging, or from localized treatment.
T3	Tumor has grown through the prostate capsule (tissue that surrounds the prostate itself) and/or into the seminal vesicles.
T4	Tumor has spread further to areas adjacent to or near the prostate, such as the bladder neck, external sphincter, levator muscles, pelvic wall, or rectum.
Regional Lymph Nodes (nodes near the prostate or within the pelvic area, N stage)	**What does this mean?**
Nx	Regional lymph nodes cannot be evaluated right now.
N0	No regional lymph nodes have cancer.
N1	Regional lymph node(s) has some cancer.
Metastatic Disease (M stage)	**What does this mean?**
Mx	Distant metastases could not be evaluated or determined right now.
M0	No distant metastases.
M1a	Non-regional (beyond the pelvic area) lymph node(s) have some cancer, either side or both sides of the body are involved.
M1b	Cancer has spread to the bone(s).
M1c	Cancer has spread to other sites or organs in the body (for example, lung or liver).

Testosterone Levels There is some preliminary research to suggest that a patient who had an abnormally low testosterone level *before* receiving an LHRH medication or surgical removal of the testicles could have a more aggressive prostate cancer, and that it may be more difficult to treat. This is preliminary, but it does make some sense that such a cancer would be able to grow with less testosterone available, making LHRH medication possibly less effective. In other words, some of these cells may have found a way to survive without much testosterone.

Time From Initial Treatment To CRPC Diagnosis If you were treated for localized prostate cancer, and then it rapidly progressed to become HRPC, this could indicate a more aggressive cancer. However, if you were diagnosed and treated for localized prostate cancer, and many years later the disease came back, and several years after that it became HRPC, it would imply a slow, steady cancer that may have a better prognosis.

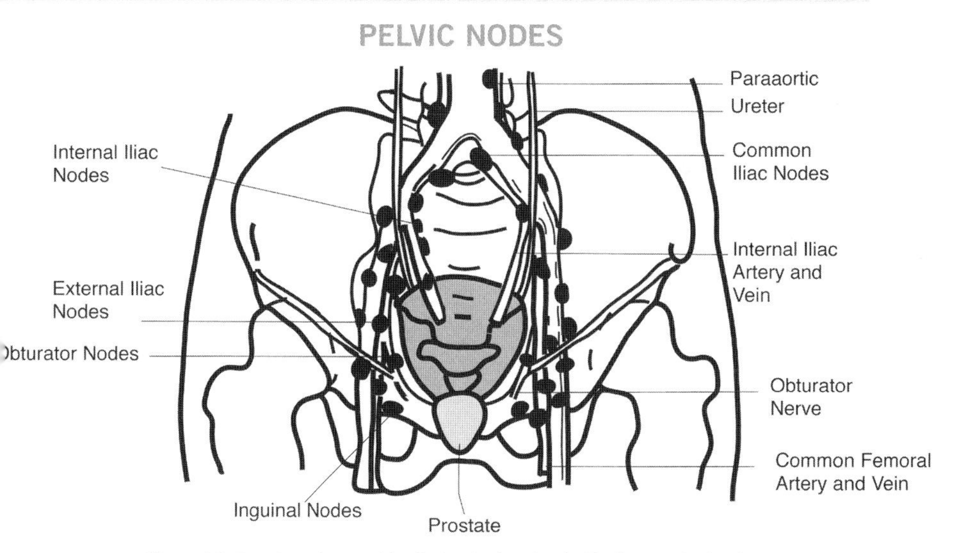

The pelvic lymph nodes are the first set of nodes in the human body where prostate cancer usually goes after growing beyond the prostate area.

Visceral Disease or Soft-tissue Disease The literal meaning of visceral is "of the internal organs," and this has come to mean cancer that has spread to locations apart from the prostate or bones, such as the liver, lungs, or other areas far from the prostate. Individuals who have visceral disease or cancer in multiple areas of the body and around the prostate tend to have a worse prognosis than those without disease in these areas. This is because the disease has advanced further. The situation is similar with what is called "soft-tissue disease," where the cancer has gone to non-bony areas such as organs and/or regional or non-regional lymph nodes.

ABDOMINAL NODES

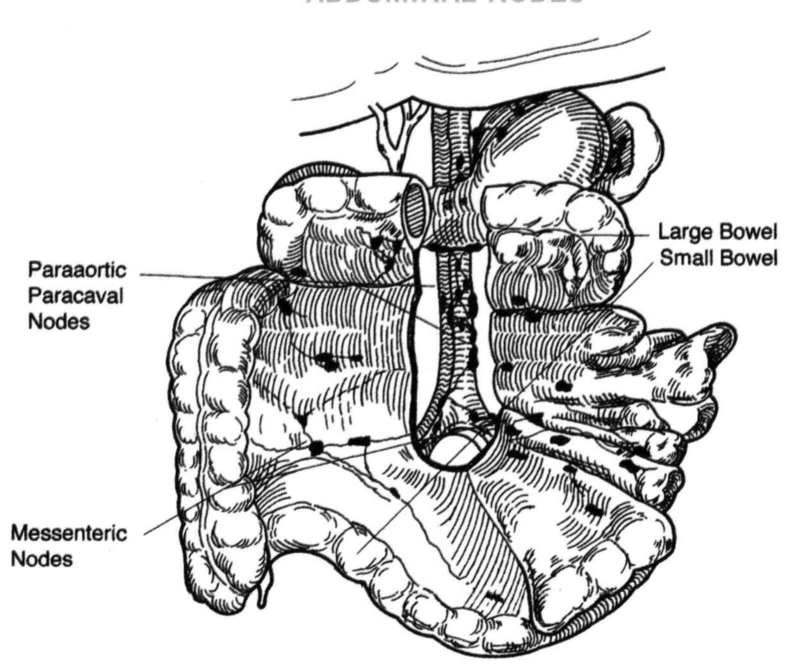

The abdominal pelvic lymph nodes are the second set of nodes where cancer may typically spread.

Volume or Amount of Cancer In general, the greater the amount of cancer in your body, the more aggressive the tumor, and the more serious the situation. For example, someone with cancer in the lymph nodes, in some organs, and in many bones tends to have a more aggressive cancer as compared to someone with just a few tumors located on a single bone. This is why working with your doctor to find the

PERI HILAR/SUPRACLAVICULAR NODES

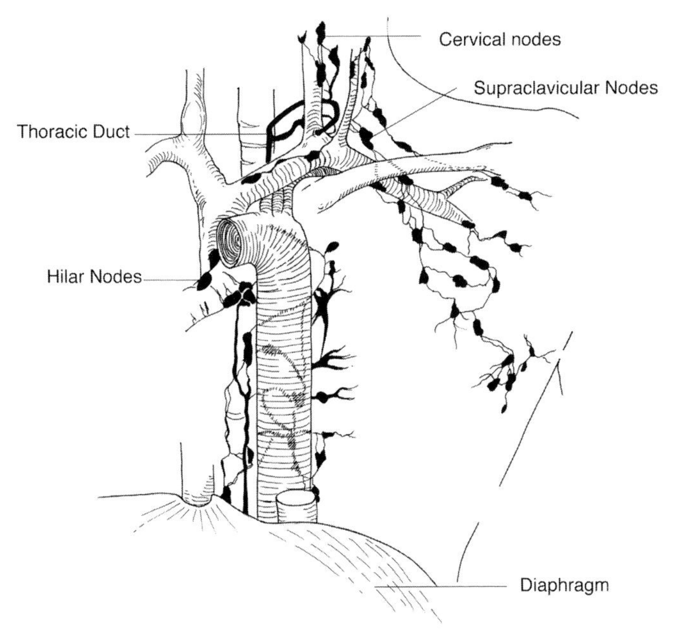

The Peri Hilar/Supraclavicular lymph nodes, located generally speaking in the chest and neck area, are usually the third set of nodes where prostate cancer spreads.

location of your tumor sites as early as possible is an important tool in planning treatment.

Weight Loss When the cancer itself is impacting a variety of areas of the body and causing extreme weight loss, this usually means that the cancer has become more aggressive and occupies more of the body as compared to someone without weight loss. In general, when men have castrate levels of testosterone because of LHRH treatment or surgery, there is usually some weight gain, or it is at least difficult to lose a lot of weight, even with exercise and diet. Therefore, when a patient begins to lose weight, this is often associated with a worse prognosis. Exceptions include when a chemotherapy drug causes nausea, resulting in weight loss due to a lack of appetite and not because the cancer is progressing. Weight loss due to cancer spread is more troubling.

Question 5: What treatments are available for my HRPC right now?

Many options currently exist, including:

- Anti-androgen addition or withdrawal
- Secondary hormonal therapies
- FDA-approved therapies
- "Off-Label" use of a drug already approved for a different type of cancer
- Enrolling in a phase-1, -2, -3, or -4 research study
- Find a drug in a phase-3 clinical trial that is available for an Early/Expanded Access Program (EAP) or Compassionate Use Program

As this book was being written, it became apparent that we would need to do a quick review of the process that drugs go through before they are readily available for use on patients. After some initial laboratory testing, it may be determined that a drug is ready for human testing. Before it receives a final approval from the FDA, it will go through several phases of testing. In the following section you'll find more information on what happens in each phase of testing and who is eligible to participate. In considering any trials, first check to see if you will be required to pay for anything for the trial. One advantage of being in such a trial, in addition to receiving a potentially exciting new treatment and contributing to research knowledge that could help you and others, is that there should be little to no cost for you. Patients also participate in clinical trials to try therapies for which they do not technically qualify under FDA guidelines. For example, a patient who does not have metastatic disease may join a trial for a drug only FDA-approved for metastatic patients thus far. Here, quickly, are the differences among phase-1, -2, -3, and -4 trials:

Phase-1 Clinical Trial

Who are the best candidates? Individuals with limited, minimal, or no treatment options.

Description:

- Generally enroll fewer than 100 patients.
- May test different types of cancers or a single type of cancer.
- Enroll a small number of participants to generally determine how a new treatment should be delivered in terms of the most effective maximum dosage, safest dosage, how often the drug should be given, and in what form the drug should be given (IV, pill, injection, patch, gel). It is not unusual for a new drug to be tested at several doses, monitoring efficacy and all side effects.

What is the catch? Drugs that have not gone beyond phase-1 testing still have many years of testing before they may be approved. The exception to this rule is a drug being tested in phase 1 that is already approved for another cancer. It then is possible to get it off-label, meaning you may have access to this drug immediately if you qualify (for financial reasons, clinical reasons, specific doctor choice, etc.), so you do not need to be in a clinical trial.

Phase-2 Clinical Trial

Who are the best candidates? Individuals who have minimal to moderate options, but who want to test a new and exciting emerging treatment.

Description:

- May enroll fewer than 100 to several hundred patients.
- Enroll a higher number of patients to begin to test the safety and efficacy of a specific dosage.
- These trials usually enroll participants with a specific type of cancer and generally test against the standard of care for an experimental treatment.

What is the catch? Drugs that have not gone beyond phase-2 testing still have several years of testing before they may be approved. The exception to this rule is a drug being tested in phase 2 that is already approved for another cancer. It then is possible to get it off-label, meaning you may have access to this drug immediately if you qualify (for financial reasons, clinical reasons, specific doctor choice, etc.), so you do not need to be in a clinical trial.

Phase-3 Clinical Trial

Who are the best candidates? All types of HRPC patients may qualify because they should (make sure you check) get the standard currently available approved treatment or one of the most promising treatments available (but not approved), involving a drug that has already done so well in phase-1 and -2 testing that it is ready to be tested in phase 3.

Description:

- Determines whether or not the promising drug will get FDA approval.
- Generally enrolls hundreds to over a thousand patients at many different locations.
- A participant is randomly assigned to the current approved treatment or the new potential treatment (a process called randomization). In other words, every participant gets the standard-of-care/approved treatment for this condition, or else gets the new and emerging potential treatment.
- "Crossover" is also usually available in a phase-3 trial. This means if you stop responding to the treatment that you are initially assigned (either the standard of care or potential drug), then you will be allowed to get the other treatment in the trial if you want it. Ask about this possibility in any clinical trial.

What is the catch? Drugs that have not completed phase-3 testing still have at least one to a few more years to be tested before they can get approved. The exception to this rule is a drug being tested in phase 3 that is already approved for another cancer. It then is possible to get it off-label, meaning you may have access to this drug immediately if you qualify (financial reasons, clinical reasons, specific doctor choice, etc.), so you do not need to be in a clinical trial.

Phase-4 Clinical Trial

Who are the best candidates? All type of HRPC patients who qualify because they should receive an approved treatment for HRPC.

Description: Involves further testing of a treatment *after* it has been approved in order to further investigate how best to continue to use this treatment.

What is the catch? Drugs that have completed successful phase-3 testing and are entering phase-4 testing have been approved, so why enter a clinical trial for a drug that is already available and probably covered by insurance? A few possible reasons are that the drug may be provided at a lower cost to you in terms of out-of-pocket expense, or that you may want to continue to support research and knowledge on an available drug, or because the new protocol with the drug being tested is one that may have a better response potential as compared to the standard of care. There are some phase-4 tests that involve getting more frequent treatments or more potentially potent dosages, and for someone with more aggressive HRPC this may be an attractive option.

Question 6: What is "early/expanded access" or "compassionate use," and why is it important to some men with HRPC?

Answer: Individuals with few or no remaining treatment options or those who are no longer responding to any of the currently available treatment options for HRPC may be given access to phase-3 drugs at little to no cost. Efforts are currently underway to expand the number of drugs available to patients through this valuable program. Always be sure to ask to see if a drug is available for an interesting new treatment if you have limited options or do not qualify for the study. The potential downside is that just because a drug becomes available for EAP or Compassionate Use does not mean that it will be effective.

In upcoming chapters, we'll consider a number of currently recognized FDA-approved treatments for HRPC and drugs that are in phase-3 testing. We'll give a listing of some drugs that are approved for use in other cancers that might also be beneficial in treating HRPC (off-label drugs) and promising drugs that are in the early stages of testing. As you read those chapters, you will get more detailed information on the full scope of possible therapies to discuss with your physician to determine the best course of action for your individual situation. Following the sections on treatment, we'll spend some time discussing side effects and offer suggestions on preventing and mitigating them. Remember, an informed patient can better weigh his options and make an educated choice on treatment plans.

Notes

Notes

Three *Minimal* Treatment *Options*

Chapter Two

Here is one quick tip—you may want to be SURE that you have HRPC. You can elect to get a total testosterone test, preferably with the blood drawn in the morning when testosterone levels are generally highest. For HRPC, your blood testosterone should be less than 50 ng/dL (1.7 nmol/L). In a very small number of situations (fewer than 5 percent), a rise in PSA is not due to HRPC, but rather due to an actual rise in testosterone. In such a case, the patient is considered to have HRPC even though he did not really have it. Rather, the therapy used to reduce testosterone levels was not able to completely get into the blood and effectively reduce testosterone to castration levels.

After establishing that you do, indeed, have HRPC, there are many options you should consider, along with your physician.

Three Minimal Treatment Options for Early HRPC When the PSA rises several times while a man has castrate levels of testosterone (less than 50 ng/dL [1.7 nmol/L]), there are a few quick options that need to be considered for some patients before other options come into play.

Some men have a rising PSA on ADT, but no signs or symptoms of metastatic disease. These men have non-metastatic HRPC (PSA-only relapse), and they have a higher risk of developing cancer in the bones in the future. However, this can take many years to occur. Thus, these men do not truly qualify yet for the FDA-approved metastatic HRPC treatments. So, what to do? Treat this disease with the FDA-approved drugs, something else, or not at all? A couple of minimal approach treatment options to HRPC may be attempted before other drug treatments, namely observation (rarely used) and, more commonly, the use of a low-dose anti-androgen, followed by anti-androgen withdrawal (AAWD). At some point, more aggressive treatments, such as secondary hormonal therapies, become a better option. Keep in mind that several different secondary hormonal treatments involve multiple options that can be used by themselves, one at a time (sequentially), or, in some cases, together. More information on each of these minimal treatment options follows.

OPTION 1 Active Observation/Surveillance

Some men with a low PSA, or a PSA that takes a long time to double in number (prolonged PSA doubling time), and no signs or symptoms of metastatic disease are potential candidates for undertaking no additional treatment for a certain period of time, as long as most of these men remain on ADT and are monitored regularly by a doctor.

OPTION 2 Low-Dose Anti-Androgen Pill

Please note that this is also considered a form of secondary hormonal treatment by some physicians, especially when taking higher doses of these medications. For more information on use of a higher dose anti-androgen pill, see chapter three.

One way to remove 90 to 95 percent of male testosterone is to get an LHRH injection or an orchiectomy (surgical removal of the testicles). However, another 5 to 10 percent of testosterone is produced by the adrenal glands. One way to block the impact of that extra testosterone is to add a drug that blocks the androgen receptor (AR), simply known as an anti-androgen. There are three anti-androgens used in this situation, namely bicalutamide, flutamide, and nilutamide.

Therapy using LHRH treatment (or orchiectomy) plus an anti-androgen pill is known by several names, including combined androgen blockade (CAB), combined androgen deprivation treatment, maximum androgen blockade (MAB), and complete androgen suppression. Regardless of the name, such therapy is a simple approach to use to determine whether the PSA can be stabilized or even reduced.

In a review over a decade ago of twenty-seven randomized clinical trials for locally advanced or metastatic disease studying the benefits of ADT (LHRH) alone as compared to combined ADT (LHRH plus a low-dose anti-androgen), researchers found only a small benefit (approximately 2 or 3 percent over five years) in survival for some patients receiving the combined therapy. Thus, most anti-androgens are used when the PSA increases on ADT; using them can lower side effects and cost.

Dosage A range of low-dose anti-androgen options exists.

Advantages These drugs are simple to take. There are now some generic options, so check availability and price, please. They can have some effectiveness when given in higher doses for HRPC patients, especially when used in the early stages of HRPC (see also secondary hormonal options in chapter three). If a patient responds quickly to one non-steroidal anti-androgen, he is likely to respond to the other two after that one anti-androgen loses effectiveness.

The catch These pills are not inexpensive. Also, if the AR is blocked, the small amount of estrogen in a man's body may become more potent, so breast pain (mastalgia) and breast enlargement (gynecomastia) are not uncommon. Also, these drugs can cause sexual dysfunction and increase the risk of gastrointestinal problems, hot flashes, and liver toxicity.

What else do I need to know? It should be kept in mind that the amount of cancer is generally inversely related to the impact of the anti-androgen pill. So, men with asymptomatic, non-metastatic disease have a much greater chance of responding favorably as compared to men with symptoms and metastatic disease.

Remember, patients who respond to one anti-androgen are more likely to respond to the other two anti-androgens. Also, please keep in mind that each anti-androgen comes with some unique side effects and other concerns.

- Bicalutamide is the easiest to take and the most effective at the lowest doses, but is known for having a higher rate of breast discomfort.
- Flutamide is inexpensive, but it needs to be taken 2 to 3 times a day. It causes a higher rate of diarrhea and liver toxicity as compared to the other anti-androgens.
- Nilutamide can, in rare situations, cause impaired night vision or lung inflammation (pneumonitis).

All of the above anti-androgens can be taken one after another, or in high doses (see chapter three), or not at all after your PSA rises on LHRH injections, or after surgery to remove the testicles.

OPTION 3 Anti-Androgen Withdrawal

Cancers can develop resistance to many medications in a somewhat similar way to how bacteria develop resistance to an antibiotic. This was acknowledged in 1992 when the concept of anti-androgen withdrawal (AAWD) syndrome was first recognized. It was found that, after a period of time on treatment with an anti-androgen pill, a tumor could actually use the drug to stimulate its own growth! Simply removing the anti-androgen when the PSA increase occurs has become a form of treatment (or non-treatment, really). Because the tumor can no longer use this specific anti-androgen as fuel, the PSA goes down. A PSA drop of 50 percent when an anti-androgen is removed is classified as a true AAWD. Only about 20 percent of men see a PSA benefit when going off the anti-androgen pill, but it still seems to be worth it for those who do respond.

Dosage No dosage needed; just remove the anti-androgen pill for several weeks. In the case of bicalutamide, the pill should be discontinued for longer (4 to 6 weeks).

Advantages A patient can get a treatment effect or a PSA reduction without doing anything except removing a pill from his daily regimen. It can usually be determined whether the patient is getting a benefit from AAWD within 6 weeks.

The catch You will need more frequent PSA testing and visits to the doctor after seeing a PSA increase (while you were on an anti-androgen).

What else do I need to know? AAWD can potentially be undertaken with any anti-androgen drug.

Although these minimal treatments may work for selected patients for a time, at some point additional therapies will likely be needed to manage the HRPC. Chapter three will discuss a variety of options that are generally referred to as secondary hormonal treatments.

Notes

Secondary *Hormonal* Treatments

Chapter Three

After diagnosis with HRPC, you begin to consider a number of options with your physician. Several options exist in addition to the FDA-approved treatments for HRPC. Some of the most widely used medications for HRPC are the so-called "secondary hormonal treatments," which work in a variety of ways. Some may even work by reducing testosterone below the accepted castrate level (to nearly 0 ng/dL). Regardless of how they act, you should be aware of these options.

Many doctors and patients like these secondary hormonal options, but interestingly they have never been approved for the specific purpose of prostate cancer treatment for men with HRPC. Why? It is probably because the drugs themselves were available for years for other purposes before doctors started to try them for HRPC. When the drugs were found to be effective for prostate cancer as well as the other purposes, there was no desire to recruit patients for an official clinical trial to exactly quantify their effectiveness, although it would have been better for patients to have such an official clinical trial completed.

Each secondary hormonal therapy has its own cost considerations. Some are inexpensive (estrogen, for example), and some are more costly (such as anti-androgen pills). Because doctors will use some of these options, we'll discuss the advantages and drawbacks of each therapy. Keep in mind that a true response to a secondary hormone therapy is determined using a variety of tests, including one for PSA reduction, in the first few months of treatment (usually 3 months). The larger the response the better, for some patients. A 50 percent or more drop in PSA is outstanding, but a smaller response is also beneficial. A response to a secondary hormone treatment also may be determined using an imaging test, and even at times by considering a symptom reduction (less pain, for example). You can review with your doctor to determine whether a particular treatment is working for you.

Question: Why are adrenal glands so important to HRPC and the secondary hormonal treatments?

Answer: *Other than the testicles, the human body makes androgens or male hormones in the adrenal glands (one of which sits on top of each kidney). The actual metabolic products that come from the adrenal gland hormones are known as "adrenal androgens," or "androgen building blocks," or "precursors" because they are used to make testosterone. Adrenal gland androgens include dehydroepiandrosterone (DHEA), dehydroepiandrosterone sulfate (DHEA-S), and androstenedione. They all have the potential to continue to stimulate prostate cancer growth. Even if a patient has castrate levels of testosterone, it is known that adrenal gland androgens can at least weakly stimulate the androgen receptor (AR).*

Thus, dietary supplements that should NOT be used when taking a secondary hormonal therapy include DHEA, DHEA-S, Tribulus Terrestis (which may have some DHEA-resembling compound in it), androstenedione, or any other supplement that claims to increase male hormone (testosterone) levels. Androstenedione is no longer sold over the counter, but there are still ways it can be obtained.

The problem with these supplements or compounds is that they can offset the impact of some of the secondary hormonal therapies as the treatments work better when the body has lower levels of these compounds. For example, new studies have shown better responses to anti-androgen drugs in individuals with lower DHEA blood levels. Therefore, be watchful for those compounds in supplements, and be sure always to check with your physician before taking a supplement.

CORTICOSTEROIDS

Corticosteroids are not considered to be true "secondary hormonal treatments" like the other drugs listed in this chapter. However, they are often given in conjunction with these drugs as well as a number of other HRPC treatments, so some information is being offered on them here.

Also known as glucocorticoids (generally); examples include: dexamethasone, hydrocortisone, prednisone, prednisolone, and methylprednisolone.

How is it taken? Usually as a pill, but can also be given by injection or intravenously (IV).

Dosage There is a variety of drugs and doses. It is not unusual to see patients taking 30 to 40 mg of hydrocortisone, or 10 mg or less of prednisone, or less than 1 mg of dexamethasone. Doctors are careful about the potency of these drugs.

Steroid Medication Review

Hydrocortisone—least potent
Prednisone—4 times more potent than hydrocortisone
Prednisolone—5 times more potent than hydrocortisone
Methylprednisolone—5 times more potent than hydrocortisone
Dexamethasone—most potent, 30 times more than hydrocortisone

Advantages These drugs are simple to take and have a good safety record.

The catch These drugs serve largely to reduce the side effects of some secondary hormonal drugs (ketoconazole or abiraterone) and chemotherapy drugs. They also suppress the immune system.

What else do I need to know? These medications have at least some anti-prostate cancer effect, probably by lowering adrenal androgen production. They have not received a lot of attention compared to the other secondary hormone therapies because they do not appear to be as effective or have an impact that lasts as long as the other therapies. Regardless, it is important to know that they at least have some impact. There does not seem to be an advantage to using one specific corticosteroid drug or dosage as compared to another, but check with your doctor on the latest research.

ESTROGEN

Also known as DES, estradiol, or by multiple generic names.
How is it taken? pill, patch, or injection.
Dosage Various doses based on the drug and situation.
Advantage Usually inexpensive, and it also has a role in reducing hot flashes and preventing bone loss in very small dosages.
The catch It increases the risk of several cardiovascular problems, particularly blood clots, so the drug is usually given with a prescription blood thinner. It also can cause breast pain and enlargement and fluid retention. The higher the dosage, the higher the risk of serious side effects.
What else do I need to know? The "female" hormone estrogen has been used for more than 50 years to treat prostate cancer. In some countries, it is still used to lower testosterone levels and function as an androgen deprivation treatment (ADT) instead of LHRH therapy. However, in most countries, LHRH drugs replaced estrogen many years ago because estrogen has serious cardiovascular toxicity (blood clots, edema, high blood pressure) in higher doses, especially as an oral drug.

Some doctors still use estrogen for two purposes in treating prostate cancer. First, as mentioned above, it can be used to treat side effects of ADT, such as hot flashes, bone loss, and perhaps even cognitive changes. Secondly, research has shown that estrogen can reduce adrenal androgens, and it also may directly kill some HRPC cells. Lower doses of estrogen seem to cause fewer side effects, and there are now several drugs to reduce these side effects if they still occur. For example, there are blood pressure medications, diuretic drugs, and blood thinners that can reduce the risk of most of estrogen's side effects.

Newer delivery systems make it easier for some patients to use estrogen, and they may also reduce side effects. For example, some patients use an estrogen patch (estradiol transdermal patch) to reduce hot flashes. The patch appears to reduce the risk of blood clots by bypassing the liver's ability to increase the clotting production that usually occurs when exposed to oral estrogen.

However, overall, the oral form of estrogen is still very popular as a secondary hormone treatment. One of the most popular is diethylstilbestrol or DES. This drug is quite inexpensive and is prescribed in a range of doses (less than 1 mg to 2 or 3 mg/day). Most doctors prefer patients to be on a prescription blood thinner, such as Coumadin (warfarin), to counteract the blood clotting concerns.

Other notable side effects of estrogen are breast pain (mastalgia) and breast enlargement (gynecomastia). These conditions can mostly be prevented by taking an oral (pill) dose of tamoxifen daily, or more simply by getting a dose of radiation to each breast (just once, taking seconds). Some studies suggest that oral tamoxifen daily is a little more effective at preventing breast pain and enlargement as compared to radiation, but radiation works with just a single treatment. Regardless, there are many issues to consider if you and your doctor decide that estrogen is an option for you in preventing ADT side effects or as a secondary hormonal treatment.

There are also other estrogen-derived treatments that you may hear about, and they are just as effective as DES for cancer treatment or for treating side effects. Several common ones are listed below:

- EMCYT (pill, also known as estramustine phosphate)
- Ethinyl estradiol (pill)
- Estradurin (injectable, also known as polyestradiol phosphate)
- Fosfestrol (pill)
- Vivelle-Dot and others (patch)

FIVE-ALPHA REDUCTASE INHIBITORS (5AR INHIBITORS)

Also known as 5AR inhibitors, finasteride, and dutasteride (brand name Avodart).

How is it taken? pill.

Dosage A single pill, taken daily. There are two options, namely finasteride (dosage 5 mg per day) and dutasteride (dosage 0.5 mg per day).

Advantages Easy to take, with minimal side effects. Finasteride now has a generic option, but dutasteride remains in your body for a longer time (a 5-week half-life) as compared to finasteride (an 8-hour half-life). Therefore, it is possible to take dutasteride just once a week (or simply not daily), save money, and still potentially get the same benefit.

The catch With these drugs, reductions in sex drive and overall sexual function are possible, as are breast tenderness and enlargement. Hot flashes and liver toxicity are also potential side effects. A recent large study of prostate cancer prevention regimes found that dutasteride slightly, but significantly, increased the risk of heart failure as compared to a placebo. This possible side effect needs to be further investigated to be sure that it is an actual concern.

What else do I need to know? These medications, particularly dutasteride, are receiving a lot of attention in the area of prostate cancer prevention and beyond. The drugs have been shown to reduce the risk of non-aggressive prostate cancer. There is currently a clinical trial underway using the drugs to treat active surveillance patients who do not want immediate conventional treatment for localized prostate cancer and who do not have aggressive prostate cancer.

Over the past several years, a small study of men with a rising PSA after localized prostate cancer treatment showed interesting results. These men did not have HRPC, but they were hormone sensitive and did not go on LHRH injections. Men took twice the daily dose of finasteride (10 mg total daily) and an anti-androgen (flutamide at 125 mg twice a day). They were compared to a group of men taking just flutamide. The researchers found greater PSA reductions and a lower chance of disease progression in the combination group (finasteride and flutamide) as compared to those taking flutamide alone. The side effects experienced by the groups were similar. This suggests that a combination approach using the 5-alpha reductase inhibitor may be a potential option in the future, even for some men with HRPC.

HIGH DOSE ANTI-ANDROGEN REPLACEMENT

Also known as Non-steroidal anti-androgens, including bicalutamide, flutamide, and nilutamide. Steroidal anti-androgens include megesterol acetate (Megace) and cyproterone acetate (Androcur).

How is it taken? pill.

Dosage Dosages vary by drug and situation. Commonly used are bicalutamide in low to high doses (50 to 150 mg/day), flutamide (a range of doses), nilutamide (150 to 300 mg/day), and cyproterone acetate (in some countries such as Canada, 100 to 200 mg a day).

Advantages Simple to take. There are now some generic options, so check the price, please. Can have some effectiveness when given in higher doses for HRPC patients, especially when used in the early stages of HRPC. If someone responds quickly to one non-steroidal anti-androgen, he is more than likely to respond to the other two after that one anti-androgen is no longer effective.

The catch Non-steroidal anti-androgens are used for treatment of the cancer itself (in high doses) or along with other medications (LHRH), but steroidal anti-androgens are really just used today for treating side effects of ADT, such as hot flashes, and not commonly used to treat HRPC.

What else do I need to know? These drugs directly bind to and block the androgen receptor (AR).

Steroidal anti-androgens (cyproterone acetate and megesterol acetate) are known for having progesterone-like (female hormone–like) activity, which is why they are more commonly used to treat hot flashes from ADT (LHRH). They also have side-effect issues such as impact on sexual function, weight gain, fluid retention (edema), nausea, and a slight risk of blood clots. Cyproterone acetate has also been found to potentially increase the risk of heart disease.

Non-steroidal anti-androgens (bicalutamide, flutamide, and nilutamide) are more specific and selective for the AR, so there is a lower incidence of side effects. Research suggests that there is a good chance a patient will respond to an anti-androgen if he has already responded well to ADT or a previous anti-androgen.

KETOCONAZOLE

Also known as Nizoral.

How is it taken? pill.

Dosage 200 to 400 mg three times a day (a total of 600 to 1200 mg per day).

Advantages Arguably, the most popular currently available second-line hormonal treatment, and one of the most effective. Ketoconazole is also one of the least expensive drugs used to treat prostate cancer.

The catch Side effects are a concern. There have been many noted because this is also one of the best-studied secondary hormonal therapies. Side effects include: sticky skin, easy bruising, dry skin, liver toxicity, nausea and vomiting, breast enlargement and tenderness, fatigue, swelling (edema), and rash. Abiraterone may soon replace this drug (see chapter seven).

Question: How should I take my ketoconazole to make it the most effective?

Answer: *Ketoconazole is absorbed much better in an acidic environment, so individuals taking antacids or any acid-suppressive over-the-counter or prescription medicine (H2 blockers or proton pump inhibitors, for example) will have trouble absorbing these pills.*

Thus it is advised to take the pills with something acidic regardless of whether or not you are on an acid-inhibiting medication. For example, soda pop (regular or diet cola) is acidic and works well. The more popular recommendation is to take between 250 and 500 mg of ascorbic acid, also known as vitamin C, with each dosage. One word of caution is to avoid "pH neutral" or "buffered" vitamin C, as these have been formulated to be non-acidic and won't assist in absorbing ketoconazole. Please make sure you buy inexpensive "ascorbic acid" or plain old vitamin C when taking it with ketoconazole.

It should say only ascorbic acid on the ingredient label.

Also, do NOT take ketoconazole with grapefruit or grapefruit juice. Avoid other citrus and exotic fruit juices as well. Grapefruit particularly has the ability to block a protein in the gut (P-glycoprotein) and liver (CYP3A4), where approximately half of all prescription medications are metabolized. What does this mean? Consuming grapefruit (and possibly some other juices) may actually raise the level of exposure to ketoconazole in the body and cause more side effects. In addition, ketoconazole itself is similar to grapefruit in that it blocks the ability of the liver enzymes (CYP3A4) to metabolize a variety of drugs (cholesterol-lowering drugs or statins and some antibiotics, for example). This means that ketoconazole can increase your level of exposure to some other drugs (almost half of those on the market), and thereby increase your chance of side effects from them. For example, it can increase the risk of liver toxicity and muscle or joint discomfort from taking a cholesterol-lowering drug (statins). Generally speaking, you have to be careful what you eat and drink with ketoconazole. Also, you need to be mindful of what effect ketoconazole can have on other prescription medications you are currently taking.

This drug enzymatically inhibits the production of adrenal androgens, but it is not specific for adrenal androgens only, so it usually requires corticosteroid replacement to prevent adrenal problems. Often prescribed is 20 to 30 milligrams of hydrocortisone in the morning and 10 milligrams in the evening, or some variation of this regiment.

Higher androstenedione levels are predictive of a less-than-adequate response to ketoconazole, which further shows that this drug works by inhibiting adrenal androgen synthesis. Some doctors may want to measure androstenedione levels and, if they are high, consider a higher dosage, another treatment method, or another secondary hormonal treatment.

Working closely with your doctor is critical in avoiding any issues as you begin to take ketoconazole.

What else do I need to know? Ketoconazole has been used medically for a variety of purposes. It is a well-known synthetic anti-fungal drug, used to prevent skin and fungal infections (athlete's foot and ringworm) and is even effective in individuals with suppressed immune systems. It is also sold over the counter and as a simple prescription in very low doses (1 to 2 percent) as an anti-dandruff shampoo. It is sold as a topical cream and even an oral tablet.

This drug is very effective at reducing male hormone production and other hormones in the adrenal glands. It can reduce testosterone levels and thus has even been used in the past to prevent post-operative erections. Clinical research suggests that this drug is effective at killing some HRPC. Previous clinical research has suggested as many as 50 percent of men get some kind of response to this drug.

Ketoconazole accumulates or is absorbed by fatty tissue, which is one of the reasons it has more side effects as compared to newer anti-fungal medicines (fluconazole and itraconazole). However, this absorption also explains why it is more effective with cancer: because it can penetrate a lot of barriers.

The average dosage is 400 mg every 8 hours (1200 mg total for the day). However, this dosage causes a number of the side effects listed above. Other studies have demonstrated that by starting with 200 mg every 8 hours (600 mg total for the day) you can reduce the side effects, but the drug is still almost as effective.

Question: Why does it have to be taken every 8 hours?

Answer: *The drug is rapidly destroyed by the liver and, therefore, does not remain at an effective dosage in the blood for a long period of time. It is said to have a short half-life. For this reason, it must be taken at least every 8 hours to give optimal results.*

SANDOSTATIN

Also known as Somatostatin or somatostatin analogues (octreotide acetate or lanreotide).

How is it taken? Injection or IV.
Dosage Given as an injection or intravenously (IV) in a variety of dosages.
Advantages This is a new potential secondary hormonal treatment. Sandostatin is known for its lack of side effects. The only short-term notable side effects are some fatigue and diarrhea, especially during the first month of the treatment.
The catch Since it is new as a secondary hormonal treatment, the true positives and negatives of using these drugs for HRPC are not yet clear. Researchers are not sure whether it is even effective against HRPC.
What else do I need to know? This is a drug that inhibits growth hormone (GH) production. It is best known for treating children and adults who produce too much GH (known as gigantism in children and acromegaly in adults). GH itself is a drug that has been given in some anti-aging clinics, but the research supporting this hormone for anti-aging is weak. There are also possible serious long-term toxicity issues. In fact, GH is a troubling medication because it causes the release of another hormone known as insulin-like growth factor 1 (IGF1). Some research studies appear to show that higher levels of IGF1 may promote tumor growth. The fact that Sandostatin may help some with HRPC provides some support for this argument.

Some preliminary research suggests that, when a drug like Sandostatin is combined with a steroid medication (such as dexamethasone), it may allow hormone therapy to be slightly effective again for a time, or it may block IGF1 or another factor that allows a prostate cancer cell to survive. Using Sandostatin as a treatment is a new concept so, as always, talk to your doctor for the latest information on it.

Question: Is combining secondary hormonal treatments an option?

Answer: *Yes. There is now some preliminary research to suggest that secondary hormonal therapies may be better when they are given in combination. This seems to make* *sense, because each medication targets a separate anti-cancer pathway. Estrogen kills cells directly; high-dose anti-androgens block a receptor; ketoconazole reduces adrenal hormones and self-hormone production in tumors; and Sandostatin reduces the amount of a type of fuel that could promote tumor growth. Thus, it is not surprising that a few studies have shown a higher response rate in men with HRPC when the drugs are combined. There are even some new studies using secondary hormone therapies with medications such as dutasteride (5-alpha-reductase inhibitor) with ketoconazole, for example, or a bone maintenance drug (bisphosphonate) with multiple therapies. However, other studies have shown mixed results, so talk to your doctor to determine the best course of treatment for your situation.*

The next section in the book will consider HRPC treatments approved by the U.S. Food and Drug Administration (FDA). As was mentioned earlier, there are exciting new drug therapies being researched currently. Since this book was started, several new drugs have been added to the following section, demonstrating that research in HRPC is in an exciting period with many breakthroughs happening. Remember, each new drug being tested offers the promise of a new treatment option for HRPC patients.

FDA-*Approved* Therapies *for* HRPC

Zometa, Xgeva, *and Other* Bone-Protecting *Drugs*

Chapter Four

In this chapter, we'll consider the drug Zometa, which is widely recognized and used in treating HRPC, and a second bone health drug, Xgeva, that may actually work even better than Zometa for some patients. We'll also discuss briefly other drugs approved to reduce bone pain, namely samarium and strontium.

ZOMETA

Also known as zoledronic acid
How is it taken? IV
Approval status FDA approved
Company Novartis
Information www.us.zometa.com

Zometa belongs to a class of drugs called bisphosphonates that are generally prescribed for bone health. It is *not* an FDA-approved treatment for cancer, but it is an FDA-approved treatment for preventing or delaying problems associated with hormone-reducing drugs or from cancer itself, such as bone loss. Both Zometa and Xgeva can be used for patients with metastatic prostate cancer to prevent or delay a skeletal-related event (SRE).

Question: What is an SRE?

Answer: *Problems associated with cancer going into the bone are collectively referred to as skeletal-related events (SREs). There are several SREs caused by metastatic prostate cancer:*

Bone fractures *These are known as "pathologic bone fractures" of the spine (vertebral area) or non-spine areas (such as hip, leg, or wrist). The most common sites for bone fractures are the hip and upper legs, the spine, wrist, and ribs.*

Spinal cord compression *If prostate cancer gets into the backbone or spinal cord, it can create pressure and cause nerve damage. The nerves of the spinal cord control all sorts of body operations, so damage to the cord can cause problems such as pain, numbness, muscle weakness, and even bladder control issues.*

Radiation to the bone or an IV drug needed to get to the bones *When cancer penetrates the bone and causes pain, some patients need radiation delivered to that same site to reduce the bone pain and to potentially stop the tumor site from doing more damage. This is known as spot radiation. Other patients may require radioisotopes (radiopharmaceuticals), drugs given that find those tumor sites, reduce the pain, and potentially stop more damage to the tumor site.*

Surgery to the bone *If the bones become weak, damaged, or broken, they often need some type of surgery to repair the problem bone site.*

Hypercalcemia *Another SRE is a high blood level of calcium (hypercalcemia) that can occur with bone loss. However, bisphosphonates such as Zometa do a very good job of preventing this problem. In fact, this drug is now used in several non-cancer-related emergency situations, including in children when a blood level of calcium becomes high enough that it creates a life-threatening concern.*

Some of these SREs can be serious enough to change the way your cancer is treated overall, causing serious delays in treatment, changes in the treatment itself, or cessation of the treatment to alleviate the bone pain.

As mentioned earlier, Zometa has been FDA-approved to prevent or delay SREs. The drug significantly reduces the risk of all the above SREs to some degree, but has been most effective at reducing the risk of bone fractures, making it a popular osteoporosis drug in both cancer situations and general medicine. It also has been shown to have an impact on reducing bone pain long-term. Every man with HRPC should talk to his doctor about receiving this drug or another bone protecting medication.

Dosage Given intravenously (IV) in the oncology or urology office, clinic, or hospital to prevent bone loss and skeletal problems associated with HRPC. Total amount given per visit is generally 4 mg. It is used every 3 to 4 weeks in many cases, but can be used once every few months or even once a year in some rare cases. Your physician will decide the frequency of the IV infusions of this drug based on your situation.

Advantages This drug improves quality of life. It takes only 15 to 30 minutes to administer and prevents bone loss from hormone therapy (ADT). It may also prevent or delay harm to the bone that can be caused by prostate cancer that has become metastatic. The earlier Zometa is used in HRPC, the more it can do to prevent these problems.

The catch Calcium and vitamin D supplements should be used daily while on and off this medication (their dosages should be determined by a doctor). If your doctor encourages you to do some weight lifting because you have minimal or no bone disease, you should consider that as well to improve your bone health. Many men and women do not get the full bone health benefit because they do not undertake the lifestyle and dietary supplement changes that can improve the positive impact of the drug itself (see the side effects chapter for more information on bone health).

Question: What should I know about the common and not-so-common side effects of bisphosphonates?

Answer: *Most of the side effects of Zometa are mild and rare. For example, the most common side effect is a short-duration fever soon after the treatment. Other side effects include gastrointestinal problems (constipation), anemia, nausea, vomiting, loss of appetite, and thirst. A collection of flu-like symptoms can also occur (fever, chills, weakness, and muscle, bone, and joint aches) after the infusion. Eye pain, redness, sensitivity to light, and reduced vision have been noted in rare cases.*

If you have a kidney problem or an irregular heartbeat, Zometa can make it worse in some rare cases. A complete review of your current and recent medications with your doctor is important before you receive Zometa to prevent or reduce the risk of any side effects. It is very important that your doctor know if you have been taking any over-the-counter or prescription drug that can affect (reduce) your kidney function, such as: aspirin, non-steroidal anti-inflammatories (ibuprofen, naproxen, or celecoxib), diuretics, and angiotensin-converting enzyme (ACE) inhibitors for blood pressure. Your doctor needs to know if you have been taking any prescription aminoglycoside medications (used to treat some infections), because the combination of these drugs with bisphosphonates can reduce your blood calcium to abnormally low levels (hypocalcemia), causing all sorts of health issues. Some examples of aminoglycosides include: gentamycin sulfate, streptomycin sulfate, and tobramycin sulfate. Kidney function and blood levels of certain compounds (creatinine and calcium, in particular) will also be monitored over time by your doctor.

Also, if you have any dental problems or dental procedures planned for the near future, please talk to your doctor about them. Bisphosphonates are getting a lot of attention for a rare side effect known as osteonecrosis of the jaw (ONJ). This problem occurs when an upper or lower area of the teeth or jaw becomes infected, and this infection becomes difficult to cure while you are on the bisphosphonates. One way to reduce the risk of this problem is to get dental clearance or a clean bill of health from a dentist before you start a bisphosphonate drug. Also, ask your doctor if your bone imaging test indicates that you might be at higher risk for ONJ.

The majority of cases of ONJ are in patients who have been on bisphosphonate treatment for a longer duration, and commonly ONJ patients reported a previous dental procedure. If you develop any of the following symptoms, be sure to check with your physician right away:

- *Mouth or facial pain that resembles a toothache*
- *Chronic sinusitis (inflammation of the sinuses)*

- *Foul-smelling drainage in the jaw area*
- *Numbness in either the upper or lower jaw area*
- *An exposed bony area inside mouth when looking in mirror*

Although it has received a good deal of media attention, it is worth repeating that this side effect is very rare.

What else do I need to know? Although there are lots of osteoporosis drugs on the market, Zometa was the first one the FDA approved for metastatic HRPC. However, this does not mean that other osteoporosis-prevention pills are not an option for some patients to prevent bone loss.

Speaking just in terms of bisphosphonate or other osteoporosis pills available to prevent bone loss in men and women, there are medications that can be taken once a day, once a week (alendronate and risedronate, for example), twice a month (risedronate), or just once a month (ibandronate and risedronate, for example). All of them require that you take the medication on an empty stomach, sitting or standing, with a full glass of water at least 30 minutes before you eat anything. All of them have the ability to irritate your esophagus, which is why you need the glass of water to get the pill all the way down into the stomach. These pills do not absorb well with food in the stomach; hence the recommendation to take them on an empty stomach. The good news about the pills is that they allow flexibility and, unlike the IV bisphosphonates, do not require an office visit. However, for people who have issues swallowing pills and esophageal (throat) problems (such as Barrett's esophagus), or simply for most patients with HRPC and bone metastasis, these oral drugs are not as effective as intravenous Zometa. Remember, none of these pills are FDA approved for HRPC metastatic prostate cancer to reduce skeletal-related events.

Zoledronic acid (Zometa) is the most powerful bisphosphonate medication, which is probably why it is used often for HRPC. However, this powerful drug comes with powerful side effects, so always weigh the risk-to-benefit options with your doctor.

Question: How do the bisphosphonates work to promote better bone health?

Answer: *Although it doesn't appear so on an X-ray, bone is dynamic and constantly changing, breaking down and building up every second of the day. There are two types of cells that bone relies on to build healthy new bone. The osteoblasts help to build new bone and act to simply "fill in potholes on the road," so to speak. In contrast, the osteoclasts create the potholes, for good and bad reasons. In healthy bones, osteoclasts function to break down bone so that osteoblasts can put healthy bone back in areas of the bone that need repair. Bisphosphonates simply work by blocking or inhibiting the ability of osteoclasts to function. In this way, the skeleton stops losing any more bone and may even build a little new bone.*

Prostate cancer can increase the action of the osteoclasts, causing more bone breakdown, but it especially increases the tendency of the osteoblasts to build abnormally weak bone. This is why prostate cancer has been known for years as a cancer that causes osteoblastic bone disease. By reducing the ability of the osteoclasts to do an abnormal amount of damage, bisphosphonates are effective at reducing bone loss and SREs in prostate cancer patients.

Question: Why does prostate cancer tend to travel to the bones more as compared to most other body sites?

Answer: *Bone releases or produces a large number of compounds that prostate cancer is attracted to, more so than most other locations in the body. There is research ongoing to attempt to discover everything related to bones that prostate cancer finds attractive to determine whether production of these compounds can be shut off in order to fight the cancer. It is plausible that bisphosphonates and other osteoporosis drugs may work partly by shutting off the production of some of these compounds.*

Question: When prostate cancer goes into the bone, is this the same thing as "bone cancer" or "cancer of the bones"?

Answer: *No. Cancer that starts in the bone is very different. Cancer that starts in the prostate and eventually goes into the bone can be associated with minimal to major problems. There can be a single tumor at one bone site, or many tumors located in many bone sites from head to toe. The impacts of cancer that goes to the bones vary in each person.*

Question: When during the course of HRPC is it best to start Zometa or Xgeva?

Answer: *Research has demonstrated that the earlier these drugs are taken in the course of HRPC, the better the results. In fact, it is best to start the drugs before there is any cancer-related bone pain, but they still work well at most time periods. It is not usual for men to have received them or another bone-health drug before being diagnosed with HRPC. Some men are given Zometa or Xgeva the moment they start on hormone therapy for any stage of cancer. You will discuss treatment intervals with your physician. More treatments can equate to more benefit, but also can increase the risk of rarer side effects. For this reason, some experts suggest a limit of two years of treatment with Zometa as opposed to continuous use. There are clinical trials considering treatment frequency, so be aware that the timing and length of Zometa or Xgeva treatment needs to be a matter of ongoing discussion.*

Question: Do these drugs help with other types of cancer?

Answer: *Yes. These drugs have also been shown to be a benefit in breast, kidney, and lung cancers, and multiple myeloma (cancer of the immune cells of the bone marrow).*

These are also exactly the same drugs used currently by some postmenopausal women to prevent bone loss from osteoporosis, but the drug is known in this situation as Aclasta. It is given once a year. As you can see, this drug has fairly diverse application in the area of bone health.

XGEVA

Also known as Denosumab
How is it taken? injection
Approval status FDA approved for HRPC patients with bone metastases
Company Amgen (www.xgeva.com)
Advantages It is an injection usually given once every month, or less often in some cases, with a low rate of side effects. It may be usable at anytime in men with HRPC to improve bone health and reduce the risk of skeletal-related events (SREs). In a recently released phase-3 study, it beat Zometa in terms of preventing SREs, and perhaps at reducing the risk of metastatic bone disease.
The catch There seems also to be a rare increased risk of osteonecrosis of the jaw (ONJ) similar or even slightly greater to what has been observed with Zometa, and a higher risk of causing low blood calcium (hypocalcemia). Approximately 80 percent of patients with ONJ had a previous tooth removal, were using a dental appliance, or had poor oral hygiene.
What else do I need to know? Xgeva is an antibody that is injected monthly or less frequently. It basically blocks a signal that allows bone loss to occur and prevents SREs. Ask your doctor if it is available and can be used after or instead of Zometa.

Radiopharmaceutical Drugs

SAMARIUM-153

Also known as Quadramet
How is it taken? IV
Approval status FDA approved
Company EUSA-Pharma Inc.

STRONTIUM-89

Also known as Metastron
How is it taken? IV
Approval status FDA approved
Company Amersham Healthcare and AstraZeneca

Advantages Radiopharmaceutical drugs (radioactive IV drugs) are given several times over a period of weeks to months, in general. They are used to treat pain when cancer has gone into the bones. Once the drug is given, it goes through the body seeking cancerous areas and emits energy particles that kill some of the cells, so many individuals get some pain relief in the first week. The FDA-approved drugs samarium-153 and strontium-89 are available right now for some patients. Only one of these drugs can be given. They are never given in combination. In conjunction with chemotherapy, each may provide a survival benefit. Recent studies of samarium with chemotherapy should be discussed with your doctor.

The catch The side effects from these drugs result from radiation that goes into the bone and can cause blood cell production (of white blood cells and platelets) to be reduced. Less commonly, diarrhea can occur. The half-life of the drug samarium is much shorter than that of strontium; it seems to cause fewer bone marrow side effects because it emits radiation for a shorter time. Therefore, samarium has become more popular lately among some men with HRPC.

What else do I need to know? A phase-3 trial is underway using radium-223 by itself and in combination with other therapies in patients not eligible for Taxotere chemotherapy with symptomatic HRPC and bone metastasis. Other studies being completed are using samarium to potentially enhance the impacts of Taxotere. Preliminary studies suggest that this combination appears safe and may have more efficacy than Taxotere alone for some patients. Radium involves alpha radiation, which means that its radiation generally travels a shorter distance compared to beta radiation drugs (such as samarium and strontium), so the benefit-to-risk ratio may be better for patients. Regardless, all of these medications work well and are probably underused in HRPC patients with bone pain.

Other Non-Bisphosphonate Bone Health Drugs

As a final thought in this area, we should mention other bone-health drugs that are not in the bisphosphonate drug class.

There are several available, including:

- Calcitriol (pills) should not be used by most patients. It was combined with chemotherapy in a recent trial of men with HRPC. It did not improve their condition and may have even made it a little worse.
- Estrogen (see also the secondary hormonal treatments chapter), a partially effective secondary hormonal therapy, has cardiovascular side-effect issues, so it is not a popular osteoporosis drug for HRPC.
- Parathyroid hormone (PTH or Forteo, an injection) is an effective FDA-approved osteoporosis drug for men and women but is not being used in cancer patients because of a lack of research in this area.
- Strontium ranelate (pills, not FDA approved) is an effective drug used around the world, but it has not been tested enough in cancer patients. The same is true for strontium dietary supplements.
- Raloxifene (Evista, a pill) is FDA approved for osteoporosis, but not in HRPC because of a lack of research, and also because it increases the risk of blood clots.
- Toremifene (pill) is not FDA approved for prostate cancer and may increase the risk of blood clots.

The bottom line is that when it comes to HRPC, the only FDA-approved bisphosphonate drug is Zometa. The only other bone health drug that competes with Zometa for HRPC patients is Xgeva.

Notes

Provenge

Chapter Five

PROVENGE
Also known as sipuleucel-T
How is it taken? infusion
Approval status FDA approved
Company Dendreon
Information www.provenge.com

Provenge is the first FDA-approved personalized immune-boosting compound for the treatment of cancer that was shown to provide a survival benefit for patients. In clinical trials, the Provenge group lived significantly longer and had a 22.5% reduction in the risk of death compared with men in the control group. As a result, questions abound regarding this treatment. In this section, we'll try to provide answers about this groundbreaking new therapy.

Dosage As a quick overview, the Provenge treatment is accomplished by removing a small quantity of your immune cells at a blood bank or medical center. (More explanation of this process follows later in this chapter.) Those cells are then sent to the company's manufacturing facility. After two or three days, the patient returns to a doctor's office or medical center trained in this treatment to receive an infusion of the boosted cells. In the future, a cell-tracking system may allow the patient to follow his cells through the process. The entire Provenge procedure is repeated three times over a period of approximately four weeks.

Question: Who qualifies to get Provenge right now?

Answer: *The FDA has approved Provenge for men with metastatic castrate-resistant (hormone refractory) prostate cancer that is asymptomatic (without symptoms) or with minimal symptoms. Basically, if a* *patient's PSA rises 3 consecutive times on LHRH or androgen-deprivation therapy (ADT), and the doctor finds metastatic disease (bone metastasis, for example,using a bone scan), then that patient potentially qualifies. The FDA gave a fairly broad indication, which is very good for patients! More men will have this as an option in the upcoming years. All men with HRPC should talk to their doctor about whether or not they can qualify for the medication.*

Question: Do I have to remain on my hormone therapy (LHRH treatment) when I receive Provenge?

Answer: *In the clinical trials, men stayed on their hormone therapy, so it would seem wise to do the same. However, that decision will be made in consultation with your doctor.*

As discussed earlier, some believe that hormone therapy gives a slight immune boost itself in the way that it treats the disease, but others do not believe this boost exists. Those who believe a boost exists point to an increased immune reaction found at some tumor sites in men who had their prostate removed and were on LHRH treatment. Also, the thymus, a gland in the neck that helps to mature and perhaps produce some immune cells, shrinks with age and becomes less functional. However, researchers have noticed that in some patients the thymus can actually begin to grow again and become more active during hormone therapy. Of course, the low testosterone level produces many side effects, but it is important to consider that all men who were treated in the Provenge FDA-approved clinical trial had castrate testosterone levels during the trial.

Advantages The treatment is simple, has a low rate of side effects, and gives men a new option before (or even after) chemotherapy. The FDA has also offered flexibility in who receives it, making it available to men without symptoms or with minimal symptoms of HRPC who have metastatic disease.

The catch It's expensive. Total cost of treatment is in excess of $90,000. However, insurance, including Medicare, will cover most of the cost. Some patients may have to travel to another medical facility in their state or region of the country to receive it. The web site and toll-free number provided below will help in finding the location nearest you.

What else do I need to know? Since it is a fairly new treatment, information is not as widely available as for some of the other treatments. The maker, Dendreon, has opened a call center to assist patients in getting answers to questions and locating treatment centers nearby. The toll free number is 1-877-336-3736 (or 1–877–DENDREON). More information is also available on the product web site, www.provenge.com. There are many sites still doing and recruiting for clinical trials for Provenge, so ask the hot line, check the Provenge web site, or visit www.clinicaltrials.gov for more information.

There are numerous medical centers trained to administer the treatment right now, and more sites are being added. Both oncologists and urologists can provide Provenge.

Question: Can you walk me through the actual Provenge treatment process?

Answer: *While a quick overview was provided earlier, it is worth considering the treatment process in more detail.*

Step 1: The Leukapheresis Procedure (This process is sometimes also called apheresis or simply pheresis.) The name leukapheresis comes from leukos, for "white blood cells" and pheresis, for "to remove or withdraw." At a medical center or blood bank, blood is drawn from one arm through a catheter (similar to an intravenous or IV line). The blood goes through a machine that separates

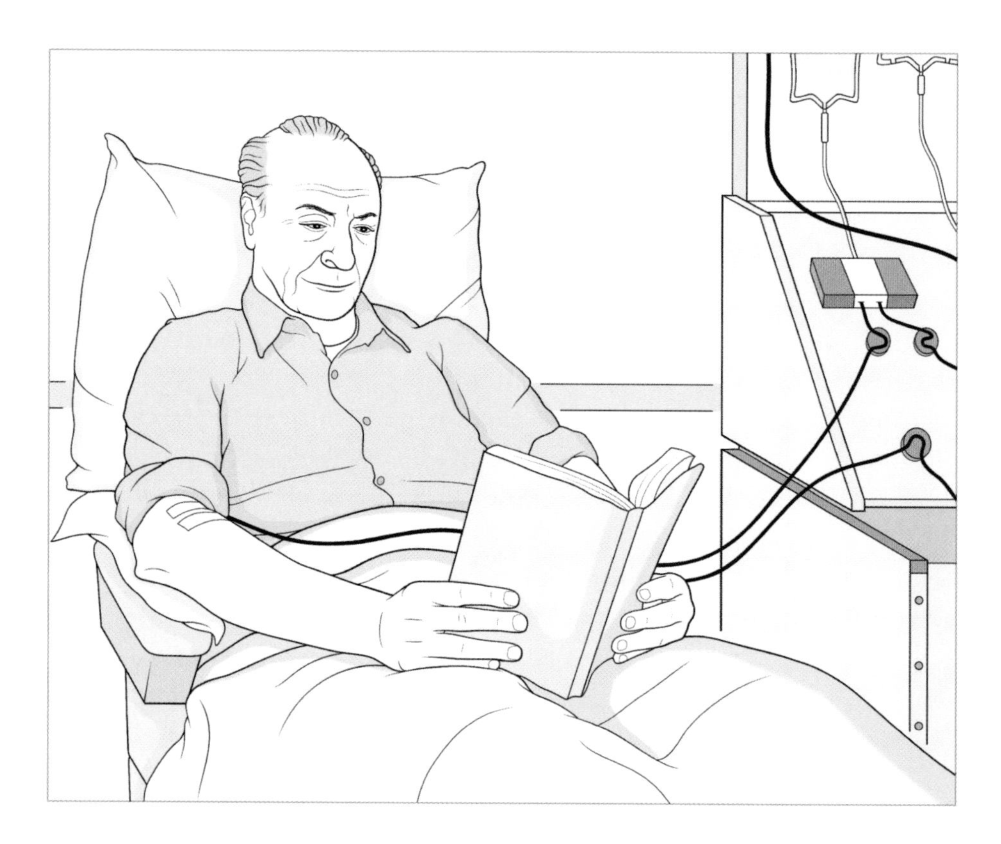

the white blood cells (immune cells) from the rest of the blood and collects them. That blood, minus some of those immune cells, is returned into the patient's other arm through another catheter. This is generally a painless procedure and involves moving only small quantities of blood out of and back into the body at any one time.

The average time for this process is about 3 hours, and the average sample size taken during leukapheresis is 8 oz (250 ml), or a cup. The collection of this cup of cells takes several hours because the immune cells need to be filtered out from the other types of cells in the blood by the machine. Patients can read or watch television to pass the time. Afterward patients can either drive themselves home or get a ride from a friend or relative, whichever they feel is best. Patients generally feel better if they come into the procedure well hydrated and do not consume any caffeine or alcohol within 24 hours of the leukapheresis, as these may contribute to dehydration. Patients may feel slightly fatigued after the procedure, but staying hydrated will help prevent this from happening. Also, try to limit excessive exercise just before and after the procedure because it will only add to the fatigue the patient may experience.

It is also important to know that at times an anticoagulant (citrate) is added to the blood in small amounts to keep cells in the machine from clumping together. Small amounts of this anticoagulant may get into your body and cause a little tingling, for example around the mouth, or even a sensation of cold or chills somewhere in the body. This is expected and should not cause concern. (See chapter nine for more information on this potential side effect.)

Leukapheresis is not a new procedure. Health-care professionals have used it in some leukemia cases for decades to remove large numbers of abnormal white blood cells that have been produced by the body in the course of the disease. Some cells, such as platelets, can be slightly reduced in number during leukapheresis, which may impact blood clotting. Rarely, a patient may experience an increased amount of bruising or easy bleeding after the leukapheresis. Step 2 occurs moments after step 1 is completed in most cases.

Step 2: The Sample Is Collected and Sent to the Manufacturing Facility The immune cells from step 1 are collected and packaged in an insulated container. They are shipped overnight to a company manufacturing facility. When a patient's immune cells arrive at the facility, they are combined with a protein that is unique to prostate cancer cells and helps to produce an eventual immune response to the patient's cancer, and another compound that helps to fully mature and boost those cells. When the cells are returned to a patient's body, they will not only help fight the tumor(s) but can also recruit other immune fighters. Now, it is time for step 3.

THE PROVENGE PROCESS

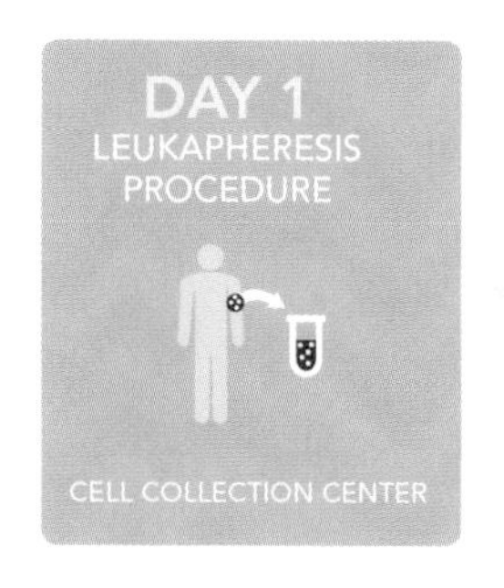

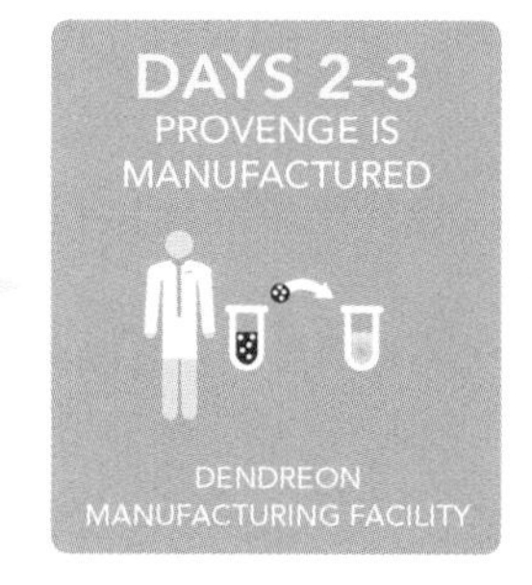

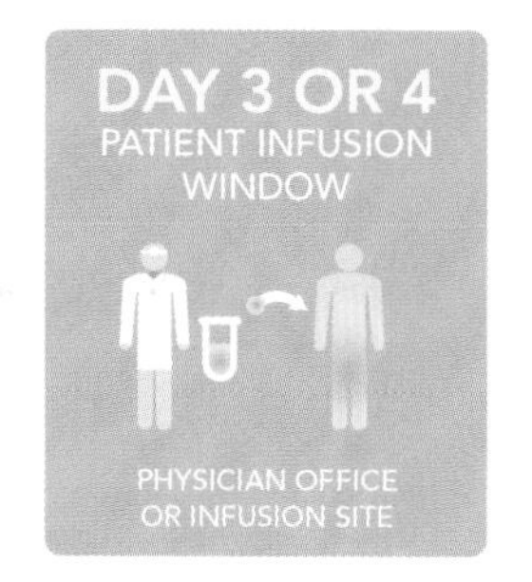

The precise mechanism of action of PROVENGE is not known.

Step 3: The Provenge Sample Is Returned to the Doctor and Infused into the Patient After 2 to 3 days, the patient's immune cells (a minimum of 50 million) have been boosted and packaged, and they are then shipped overnight to his doctor. At the doctor's office, the patient is usually given acetaminophen (Tylenol) and an antihistamine (anti-allergy) medication such as Benadryl (diphenhydramine) orally to prevent side effects. Those medications are given about 30 minutes before the actual infusion. Acetaminophen (average dose in the clinical trial was 650 mg) is effective at reducing aches and pains and fever without causing much, if any, blood thinning. Diphenhydramine (average dose in the clinical trial was 50 mg) can keep the patient's body from developing an allergic-type reaction to the infusion process. These medications are simple and excellent ways to reduce the minor flu-like symptoms that are common for a day or two after the infusion is completed. (Interestingly, the incidence of more serious, but rare, infusion reactions was greater following the second infusion [about 2 percent], and decreased to a little more than 1 percent after the third infusion.)

The patient then receives an infusion of the boosted immune cells in one arm, taking an average of one hour. The patient rests and is observed for any side effects for about 30 minutes. Patients can drive themselves home or get a ride from a friend or relative, as they prefer. The diphenhydramine (Benadryl) given may cause some drowsiness following the infusion. In the rare event that a patient does not have an accessible vein in his arm, the health-care professional can use a vein in another location, such as the neck or upper chest. The process described in steps 1 to 3 is repeated after approximately 2 weeks, and then completed a third time about 2 more weeks after that.

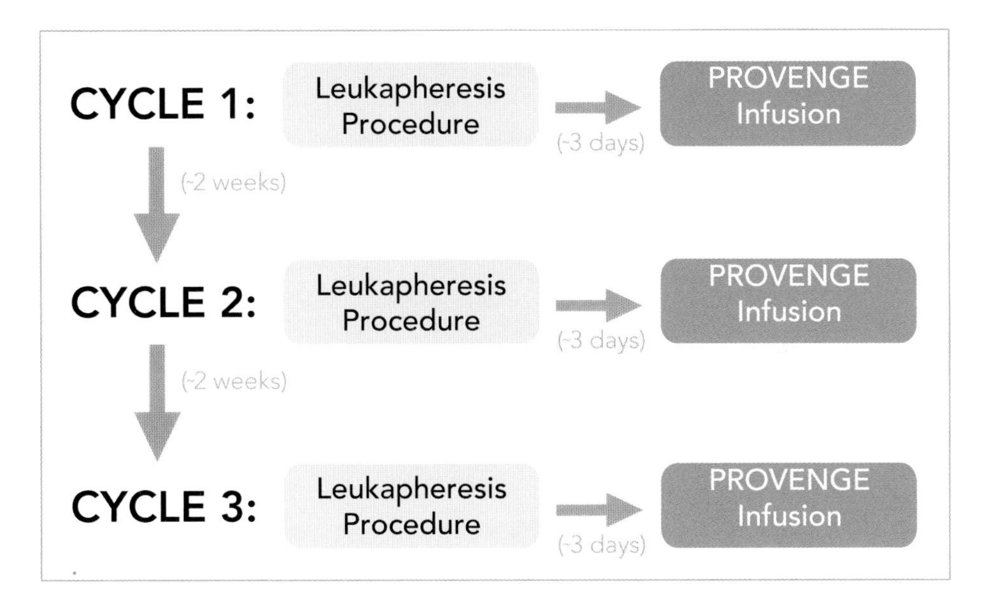

Question: What happens if a treatment is missed or delayed?

Answer: *During the clinical trials, delays in treatment did occur for a number of reasons. Once step 1 is completed, it is important to stay on schedule through step 3 unless there is a true emergency situation. If the infusion step is delayed, then the cells will not be usable and the leukapheresis would need to be repeated, adding additional cost in the case of patient delays not related to patient health. The boosting process was really the key treatment step that significantly increased life expectancy in men with HRPC.*

It is less critical that the treatments occur at 2-week intervals. Each time a treatment occurs, the patient receives an immune response that lasts for a variable but lengthy time period. The schedule developed is believed to be optimal, but patients will still receive a benefit from delayed treatments if the patient's situation requires the delay.

A good analogy for the immune-boosting process would be a military one. The patient's immune cells are basically immature inexperienced soldiers, and some are removed from the war (the body) in step 1. The immune-cell soldiers are sent to boot camp (the manufacturing facility). Within a few days, they are turned into experienced, smarter, and more fit military veterans, capable of doing battle with the cancer (step 2). Step 3 returns them to the battlefield (the infusion process) to fight the enemy, cancer.

Question: Can you explain more about the negatives associated with this treatment, other than the cost? What were some of the most common side effects, how serious are they, and how long did they last?

Answer: *The most common side effects that occur within one day after step 3 are (as reported by the* New England Journal of Medicine*):*

Chills	51 percent of the individuals
Fever	23 percent
Fatigue	16 percent
Nausea	14 percent
Headache	11 percent

Most of these flu-like side effects are temporary and are common with immune-related procedures. The side effects generally end within a day or two after the procedure. There were very few cases of "dropouts" or patients who discontinued the entire treatment because of side effects. In fact, in fewer than 1 percent of cases were any side effects serious enough to stop a patient from receiving all 3 treatments.

There are some reports of uncommon side effects,

such as constipation or diarrhea, hot flashes, muscle and joint pains, and muscle spasms. As mentioned earlier, some patients report being sensitive to citrate, the anticoagulant mentioned in step 1.

Patients should notify their doctors immediately if they have any breathing problems, chest pains, rapid or irregular heartbeats, dizziness, nausea, or vomiting, because these could signal a heart or lung problem. Also, the doctor should be notified if the patient has a fever over 100 degrees Fahrenheit, or pain or redness at the infusion or another site.

It should also be kept in mind that, although there was a low rate of serious side effects in the definitive clinical trial, there was a slightly higher percentage of cerebrovascular events, such as strokes (2.4 percent of the patients getting Provenge as compared to 1.8 percent in the control group). Statistically this was an insignificant difference and the FDA has not required a warning on the drug label. The just over a half of a percent-higher rate of cerebrovascular events could have been by chance, or it could be a result of the drug itself.

By the way, situations like this one show why safety is aggressively monitored after the approval of any new drugs so that soon there can be an update on which side effects are and are not caused by that drug. Talk to your doctor and check the drug's web site for ongoing side effect updates or any concerns about stroke. It is always important to review the latest information on side effects before starting any treatment.

Question: Are older patients (65 years and older) more likely to experience a side effect from Provenge as compared to younger patients?

Answer: *No. There were no differences in safety between older and younger men. The latest Provenge clinical trial included men as young as 40 years old* *and as old as 91 years old, with the median age in the study being 71 years old. Approximately 90 percent of men in the clinical trials were Caucasian, 6 percent African American, and the remainder of other races, so a definitive statement on the impact of Provenge on minority populations/races cannot be made at this time.*

Since this treatment works in a new and different way, it is worth considering how doctors know that patients are responding to Provenge. Only in a minority of patients is there a PSA drop or a change in an imaging test, such as a bone scan. The FDA no longer bases its evaluation of response in clinical trials for men with HRPC on a change in PSA, but rather on the extension of life. This FDA evaluation change makes a great deal of sense due to the fact that therapies may not change PSA, but may still extend life. This is what was demonstrated in the Provenge clinical trials. Provenge extended survival in patients with HRPC significantly more than the control group and therefore was approved by the FDA for treating HRPC patients.

There was a median survival benefit of 4.1 months. This means that half the patients taking Provenge survived longer than that time and half shorter. About a third of the men in the latest clinical trial were still alive 3 years after treatment! Provenge was found to be an effective treatment, coupled with a low incidence of side effects,. While nothing less than a cure is a true "breakthrough," extending survival continues to open up new treatment methods under development to HRPC patients.

One possibility that is sure to get additional study in the future is whether patients would benefit from a "booster" Provenge treatment at a later time. One early study seems to indicate that a Provenge booster may increase PSA doubling times in certain patients. It is fair to say that research on this possibility may be in the news in the future.

Question: What about using Provenge with other treatments, such as before or after chemotherapy or with bisphosphonates?

Answer: *A notable percentage of men from the clinical trial (20 percent) had already received chemotherapy when they were treated with Provenge, so it would be expected that some chemotherapy patients would also qualify for Provenge. An interesting analysis from a previous clinical trial found that men seemed to have significantly prolonged their lives on chemotherapy (Taxotere or docetaxel) if they had received Provenge before the chemotherapy. Thus it seems Provenge may have improved the efficacy of a later treatment. This will certainly get more research going forward.*

In the Provenge IMPACT clinical study, almost half (48 percent) of the men were on osteoporosis drugs when the study started. Therefore, Provenge can be given in men who are or are not on these medications.

The biggest concern may be getting chemotherapy and/or prescription steroid medications just before starting Provenge treatment. Because these medications can theoretically reduce the immune response of Provenge, patients should avoid steroid use within 28 days or chemotherapy within 3 months of starting Provenge treatment.

Question: What if I have HRPC and there is no cancer in my bones, but there is some cancer in my lymph nodes. Would I still be able to receive Provenge?

Answer: *Since a small percentage of men with HRPC in the Provenge clinical trials had cancer only in their lymph nodes, insurance should cover some men in this situation, allowing them to receive Provenge. However, there are many men with prostate cancer who have cancer in their lymph nodes, but some are still sensitive to androgen-suppression therapy and/or radiation. These* *men do not have HRPC, which means they would not be eligible to receive Provenge at this time.*

Worth considering in this section are any diet or dietary supplements that would benefit patients undergoing Provenge treatment. Generally speaking, "less is more" during this treatment. In other words, Provenge patients should not take any supplement that says it is an "immune booster" or "immune modulator," or that makes claims to "support the immune system." Theoretically, such supplements could block or disrupt the action of Provenge, so why take that chance?

Overall, what is good for your heart is also good for your immune system. If you think about all the things in diet and life that are heart healthy, almost all of them turn out to be immune-healthy recommendations, or help make your immune system as healthy as possible. Check the section later in the book for more information on heart-healthy diet and supplements, but here are a few quick suggestions pertaining to your immune system:

Tip 1: Alcohol Moderate to slightly higher-than-moderate levels of alcohol intake from any source (beer, hard liquor, or wine) on a regular basis can reduce the effectiveness of your immune system.

Tip 2: Blood Pressure and Cholesterol High blood pressure (hypertension) that is not under control and high cholesterol can lead to immune problems and make heart disease worse.

Tip 3: Blood Sugar High glucose (sugar) and other abnormal health numbers (hemoglobin A1c) could compromise your immune system.

Tip 4: Dental Disease An unhealthy mouth can cause bacteria and other organisms to travel to other body sites, stressing the immune system.

Tip 5: Diet Heart-healthy diets (such as the Mediterranean diet, for example) are immune healthy, but this also implies that heart-unhealthy diets are immune-unhealthy diets.

Tip 6: Environment Regular exposure to some pollutants, such as lead and exhaust fumes, can reduce your immune function.

Tip 7: Medications Some pills or injections (for severe arthritis, for example, or for autoimmune disease, or even for severe allergies) work by reducing the effectiveness of your immune system, so review with your doctor any medications that might inhibit the impact of Provenge. Note: Diphenhydramine (Benadryl) is given only before each Provenge infusion, but this drug has a minor, temporary, and specific immune-reducing effect (to reduce side effects of the infusion itself), so this is no problem.

Tip 8: Exercise Moderate, regular exercise is healthy, but extreme exercise (daily triathlon training, for example) can cause immune suppression.

Tip 9: Sleep Reducing sleep by even a few hours can cause immune suppression. Naps and regular sleeping hours should be encouraged.

Tip 10: Tobacco Smoke causes large nutrient reductions in the blood. Immune cells rely on some of these key nutrients for activity, so stay away from smokers, smoking, and smokeless tobacco.

Tip 11: Stress Large quantities of immune-suppressing hormones are released with stress, so try to monitor your stress levels. If you need help with your stress levels, talk to your doctor or caregiver about this.

Tip 12: Vaccinations Ask your doctor whether you are up to date with your vaccinations, and which ones (if any) you qualify for at this time. For example, research has shown that if you qualify for a flu shot and get it, it may provide other less obvious benefits for you. The shot may reduce your risk of other diseases (cardiovascular) and infections while your immune system is being challenged by other things.

Tip 13 and 14: Weight and Waist Higher body weight, body mass index (BMI), and especially belly fat increases over a short period of time can overstimulate the immune system and direct it toward the fat tissue as opposed to more important things, such as an infection or another condition.

QUESTION: What about vitamin D supplements? I hear they are good for the immune system.

ANSWER: *Vitamin D supplements are really misunderstood. They are given credit as "immune boosters" when in reality they are immune regulators. Vitamin D functions as a "thermostat" for your immune system, keeping it from over- and underreacting. Research shows that a normal blood level of vitamin D may reduce your risk of catching colds, flu, or other infections. There is also research to suggest it may prevent autoimmune disease (from an overactive immune system).*

However, care should be used in taking vitamin D. Generally, you should not supplement with more than 1000 IU per day unless you have had a 25-OH vitamin D blood test that demonstrates that you need to increase your vitamin D intake. A normal vitamin D level is between 30 ng/ml (75 nmol/L) and 40 ng/ml (100 nmol/L). A vitamin D blood level in this range is just right; it has been associated with the most clinical benefit overall (bone, heart and immune health) and no documented toxicity.

Extremely high doses of vitamin D (or any vitamin or mineral, for that matter) are not a good thing as excessive doses of products generally always cause bad side effects. For our purposes here, "less is more" is a good practice to follow.

QUESTION: Considering that Provenge is called a "vaccine" by some individuals, will this immune therapy work better in individuals without any disease or with minimal disease?

ANSWER: *Provenge is indeed being tested on men with earlier stage prostate cancer. A past trial looked at combining the popular cancer drug bevacizumab (Avastin) with the standard 3 doses of Provenge over 4 weeks, and there seemed to be a good immune response in men with a rising PSA after localized prostate cancer therapy. An ongoing clinical trial designed to test Provenge in men several weeks before surgical removal of the prostate to determine whether they get an extra benefit is being completed now. Finally, there is also a trial starting soon for men who are under active surveillance or at high risk for getting prostate cancer. Stay tuned, because this research and the research with other investigational therapies are exciting. The greatest hope for any immune therapy that works for advanced cancer is that it can work earlier in the course of the disease, to either enhance conventional treatments or be used as a treatment by itself.*

Taxotere

Chapter Six

TAXOTERE

Also known as docetaxel
How is it taken? IV
Approval status FDA approved
Company Sanofi-Aventis
Information www.taxotere.com

Taxotere is somewhat similar to an older popular chemotherapy drug, Taxol (paclitaxel), which comes from an extract of the Pacific Yew tree. However, that tree is scarce. Taxotere comes from the more abundant European Yew tree. The slight change in chemical structure at two specific points has made this drug more water soluble and potentially more effective. Some experts consider it a natural chemotherapy medicine, but others would call it semi-natural because it has been slightly altered from its origins.

It is thought that Taxotere works in several ways. It seems to cause some cancer cells to self-destruct. However, Taxotere's primary way of killing cancer cells is by targeting and interfering with cell division so that cancer cannot rapidly reproduce and grow. As such, it has an effect on the most rapidly growing cells of the cancer.

Unfortunately, the chemotherapy drug cannot discriminate between the rapidly growing cancer cells and normal cells of the human body. Therefore, rapidly dividing and growing human body cells are the ones most impacted by side effects. For example, hair, nails, gastrointestinal, and bone marrow cells (the source of white and red blood cells and platelets) grow relatively rapidly, and side effects from Taxotere have a greater chance of occurring in these areas of the body. It follows that hair loss, nausea, and a low blood cell count are common during Taxotere treatment.

Dosage Taxotere is commonly given intravenously in a dosage of 75 mg/m2 once every 3 weeks, combined with a 5-mg oral prednisone pill taken twice a day. Some doctors use a different steroid besides prednisone when needed. Although this dosage is considered ideal based on clinical trials, some physicians may slightly alter it to best fit your individual needs and situation.

Advantages This is the first chemotherapy drug to demonstrate that it significantly improves the chance of living longer for men with HRPC. Results from two large phase-3 clinical trials demonstrated this and reported their results in 2004. This drug also significantly reduces pain and improves the quality of life for many patients. Many individuals miss these important points when considering the long list of potential side effects associated with Taxotere. Despite this risk of side effects, most were not serious, and not all patients experienced them. For many, many patients, the overall benefits exceeded the negatives caused by side effects. Oncologists have a lot of experience with Taxotere because it has been approved to treat many cancers over the years. Also, most of the costs should be covered by insurance.

Question: What was learned in the clinical studies that will possibly affect my HRPC treatment?

Answer: *Several results of the studies are used to help guide treatment for patients today.*

- *Researchers studied the effects of taking Taxotere (plus prednisone) every week at a lower dosage in some patients, and every three weeks at a higher dosage in other patients. It was learned that patients receiving a dosage of 75 mg/m2 once every three weeks experienced a significant survival benefit. Both groups received a quality-of-life benefit and pain reduction, but only the every-three-weeks group received a survival benefit. Treatment with 75 mg/m2 of Taxotere (plus prednisone) has become the most widely used chemotherapy for HRPC.*
- *It was noted that several criteria increased the survival benefit even more than what was normally*

experienced by patients on Taxotere. They are:
- *Lower PSA*
- *No visceral cancer (cancer in the liver or lungs, for example)*
- *Little or minimal pain*
- *Lower Gleason score*
- *Higher Performance Score (see chapter one) or FACT-P Score (an indicator of better overall health)*

Age did not have an affect on the survival benefit. Generally, the healthier the patient is at the time of Taxotere treatment, the greater the chance that he will benefit.

- *One study combined Taxotere treatment with an oral drug, estramustine (an estrogenic drug that may also impact cell division), and a steroid. While experiencing a similar survival benefit, the patients in this study didn't receive a reduction in bone pain, and serious side effects (such as cardiac, gastrointestinal, or fever issues from a low white blood count) were more common. As a result, estramustine is an option only for certain patients.*

The catch Survival is improved by a few months (2.5 to 2.9 months). However, this is a median value only, which means that approximately 19 percent of men were still alive more than 3 years after starting Taxotere. Significant side effects (such as hair loss, fatigue, and nausea) associated with Taxotere may be long-occurring and diverse, but only some patients experienced these, and most of them were considered mild to moderate in nature. However, 32 percent of patients experienced grade 3 or 4 neutropenia (immune cell reduction).

Question: I've read on the Internet about the possibility of a "PSA flare" while on Taxotere treatment. What does that mean?

Answer: *It is not unusual in a number of other cancers (breast, colon, and testicular, for example) to see tumor* *markers initially increase when treatment is started, due to release of the markers as cancer cells die or normal cells are being injured. This may be an indication that the treatment is actually working in some men. Recent studies have suggested that a small number of men receiving Taxotere for prostate cancer may also see an initial rise in PSA (in some cases more than 10 points, or, in rare cases, as much as 400 percent). This flare has no impact on the treatment duration or overall effect of the treatment. Troubling as it may seem, 10 percent or more of patients receiving the treatment may experience an initial flare in PSA. Experts suggest that at least 2 cycles (6 weeks) or more of treatment should be given to determine whether an increase in PSA means that the chemotherapy is not working (the disease is progressing) or that the increase is occurring only because the drug is beginning to work.*

What else do I need to know? Any patient with HRPC can qualify for Taxotere chemotherapy. Both Taxotere and Provenge help treat HRPC, but they work differently, so both can benefit you. Some patients will want to try Provenge first and receive Taxotere at some future point. The consideration here is that Provenge is approved for HRPC patients who have few or very minimal symptoms, and it works in cojunction with your immune system. Taxotere has helped those with more than minimal symptoms, and preliminary research suggests it may work even better if Taxotere is given at some point after Provenge. Taxotere can also suppress the immune system, so physicians will often suggest Provenge first followed by Taxotere.

Question: Can I also receive a bone health drug such as Zometa or Xgeva before or after Taxotere?

Answer: *Yes! Most men have already taken a bone drug before Taxotere is given, but there are always exceptions.*

Some men have even received bone drugs while they are receiving Taxotere.

In most circumstances an oncologist will give Taxotere and monitor your side effects. There are rare exceptions, but oncologists are the most qualified to deliver chemotherapy and treat its side effects because they have the most experience with these treatments.

Question: Do I have to remain on my hormone therapy (LHRH or ADT) when I receive Taxotere?

Answer: *In the clinical trials, men stayed on their hormone therapy (LHRH, for example), so it would seem wise to do the same. However, you should discuss this with your doctor. Some believe that hormone therapy gives a slight immune boost itself in the way that it treats the disease, but others do not believe this. As we discussed in the chapter on Provenge, the thymus gland may become more active during hormone therapy and provide patients with an immune boost. It is worth considering with your doctor the possible benefits and side effects of hormone therapy in conjunction with Taxotere.*

Question: : If I am on an anti-androgen pill, what should I do before I start Taxotere?

Answer: *This will be decided with your doctor, but, in the large clinical trial of Taxotere, men who had a rising PSA while being on an anti-androgen pill discontinued that pill before starting chemotherapy. Before beginning Taxotere treatment, men were taken off the pill for 4 weeks in the case of flutamide and nilutamide, and 6 weeks for bicalutamide, as this drug remains in the body longer than the other pills. Specific treatment plans should be discussed with your doctor.*

In general, Taxotere treatment plans vary and should be discussed with your doctor. Some patients receive many treatments of Taxotere, and some receive fewer. For example, in past clinical trials, about half of the men received 10 cycles or more of treatment, while others received fewer. Commonly, one cycle is a single dose of Taxotere given one day within a 3-week period. Therefore, 10 cycles means 10 doses over a 30-week period. How many treatments you should receive depends on how your specific cancer is responding to the medication and how well you are tolerating the side effects. Some men take a break during treatment, and others get the drug every 3 weeks as long as they are responding.

In the most famous Taxotere study that helped result in FDA approval of the drug, only 12 percent of patients needed to have their drug dose reduced at some time. However, almost 25 percent of patients had one or more treatments delayed for one reason or another. In other words, there is lots of flexibility for doctors when delivering Taxotere. If it is not given every 3 weeks for any reason, there are other doses and schedules potentially available. Commonly, most patients do well enough to receive it every 3 weeks.

An infusion or treatment of Taxotere generally takes about one hour on average. The amount of the actual chemotherapy drug is tailored to your body size. This maximizes the effect of the drug and attempts to minimize the side effects. It makes sense that larger and heavier individuals receive more of the drug than smaller, lighter patients.

Using your height and weight, the medical staff determines your body surface area (BSA), in square meters. Next, the medical staff multiplies the suggested drug dose to be given by your body surface area. For example, if your body surface area is 1.70 square meters and the dose of Taxotere to be given is 75 mg/m2, the medical team multiplies 75 x 1.70 to get 127.5 mg. If the body surface area is 2.0 square meters then the medical team multiplies 75 x 2.0 to get 150 mg. So, if two people weigh the same, the taller one will have more body surface area and will get more of the drug. Likewise, if two people are the same height, the heavier one will have more body surface area and will get more of the drug.

Question: Do I have to receive chemotherapy through the same vein every 3 weeks? That seems like a lot of needle sticks, doesn't it?

Answer: *In chemotherapy, your doctor may also have the option of implanting a catheter or "port." These are surgically placed in a larger vein in the upper body and simply stay in place for a long period of time with minimal discomfort. The port is just connected to the infusion material so that needle sticks are eliminated. The port allows you to carry on all your daily activities and makes receiving chemotherapy on a regular basis a lot easier.*

We mentioned the side effects of Taxotere treatment. Following is a list of some of the possible ones. Please keep in mind that it may be possible to prevent or treat the side effects if they do occur in your case. We'll consider them in more depth in chapter 9, on side effects, so look for more information there.

Hair loss	65 percent
Fatigue	53 percent overall, 5 percent more severe
Nausea and/or vomiting	42 percent
Low white blood count	32 percent
Diarrhea	32 percent
Nail Changes	30 percent
Sensory loss	30 percent
Inflammation of the mouth	20 percent
Swelling	19 percent
Change in taste	18 percent
Shortness of breath	15 percent
Eye tearing	10 percent

Most of these side effects were mild to moderate. Some last a day and others last months or longer (such as hair loss or fatigue). It is important to keep in mind that not all of these side effects are the result of Taxotere, but also may result because men have low levels of testosterone in general with HRPC. For example, a low level of testosterone by itself can result in fatigue.

Question: Which Taxotere side effects had a higher chance of becoming severe or life-threatening?

Answer: *A treatment-related death occurs in less than one percent of patients (about 0.3 percent) with Taxotere. However, neutropenia (a low white blood cell count of a certain type) and fatigue had a higher risk of being severe or life-threatening, as compared to other side effects. Keep in mind that both of these side effects have treatments available for them. Talk to your doctor and see the side effects chapter.*

As the chapter on Taxotere concludes, it is important to emphasize a few facts based on the large studies done on the treatment. Taxotere combined with prednisone (or another steroid drug) has become the gold-standard, first-line, primary chemotherapy treatment for men with HRPC. However, these studies also showed that using estramustine (Emcyt) could still be an option in some patients, either with or without chemotherapy. In fact, 19 percent of the men in the study had already received estramustine.

Question: Is Taxotere being tested for men with earlier stages of prostate cancer or for men with aggressive disease who do not have HRPC?

Answer: *This testing is actually underway. In other cancers, effective chemotherapy regimens have shown some benefit when this is done. However, because of the side effects with Taxotere, doctors are trying to use it for patients at the highest risk of having their cancer spread* *after localized or locally advanced prostate cancer. Thus far, the drug has not been able to extend the time during which men respond to ADT (before they become hormone-refractory). However, data will be available soon to see whether it may improve survival in this and other situations.*

Question: Has the FDA approved Taxotere for use on other cancers?

Answer: *Yes. Taxotere is used for breast cancer (some types of operable node-positive or metastatic breast cancer), gastric cancer, head and neck cancer, and lung cancer (there are two different scenarios for non–small cell lung cancer). It is also currently being tested with other cancers.*

Question: I came across the name of the drug mitoxantrone. What is its current use in HRPC treatment?

Answer: *Mitoxantrone (also known as Novantrone) was one of the first medications approved by the FDA in 1996 for HRPC treatment. It did not improve survival, but it did improve quality of life by reducing pain. Since that time, both Taxotere and Jevtana have been FDA approved for HRPC because they demonstrated a survival benefit. Therefore, the use of mitoxantrone is limited today. Officially, it is still considered a potential alternative treatment option for some HRPC patients, but generally other treatments are used to improve survival. Mitoxantrone does have side effects, including reduced blood counts, fever, nausea, and possibly an increased risk of cardiac problems such as congestive heart failure (CHF) in some patients. Talk to your doctor about the pros and cons of this drug. Its future use will probably be very limited because there are so many other drugs that can now provide more benefit to men with HRPC.*

Jevtana *and* Abiraterone

Chapter Seven

These two new drugs are the most recent additions for HRPC treatment. They are considered second-line chemotherapies and are given to treat prostate cancer that does not respond to Taxotere. Both have been shown to prolong survival in HRPC patients.

JEVTANA

Also known as carbazitaxel
How is it taken? IV
Approval status FDA approved
Company Sanofi-Aventis
Information www.jevtana.com

Jevtana is manufactured by the same company as Taxotere. It is approved to treat prostate cancer that does not respond to Taxotere. It was shown to prolong survival for those patients by an average of 10 weeks. Like Taxotere, Jevtana is used in combination with the steroid prednisone. Side effects of the new treatment include a decline in white blood cells, anemia, low platelet counts, fatigue, nausea, vomiting, infections, and kidney failure.
Dosage 25 mg/m2, once every 3 weeks.
Advantages In the clinical trial, it significantly improved survival in men with HRPC. Men had a 30 percent improvement in survival with this drug as compared to mitoxantrone (Novantrone), which translates to an increase in median survival of about 2.4 months. As we've mentioned earlier, many patients survive significantly longer than this median measurement.
The catch The rate of grade-3 or higher side effects was greater for Jevtana, as compared to mitoxantrone. As mentioned earlier, the most common side effects were a low white blood count (neutropenia), diarrhea, fatigue, and weakness.
What else do I need to know? The clinical trial included 755 patients in 26 countries who had HRPC that continued to

progress after treatment with Taxotere and androgen deprivation treatment (ADT). All patients in the study received 10 mg of prednisone per day along with either 10 cycles of carbazitaxel (25 mg/m2) every 3 weeks or mitoxantrone (12 mg/m2) every 3 weeks. It is possible that this chemotherapy drug could work as well or even better than Taxotere so that is being tested currently.

ABIRATERONE

Also known as Abiraterone acetate
How is it taken? pill
Approval status successful phase-3 trial
Company Johnson & Johnson
Compassionate use available: yes

Advantages It is a pill with a low rate of side effects, and it may be usable before or after chemotherapy. This drug has shown a proven benefit for patients who have failed Taxotere therapy and who no longer respond to or cannot take the secondary hormonal treatment ketoconazole.
The catch Abiraterone is a new treatment. A compassionate use program has been established, and patients may be able to get the drug if they are in clinical trials. Whether or not this drug works better than ketoconazole remains to be seen, but initially it appears to be safer and potentially more effective.
What else do I need to know? This is really a secondary hormone therapy that targets the adrenal areas more specifically than other drugs in this class (ketoconazole, for example) so that hydrocortisone does not necessarily always need to be given along with it. Abiraterone is known as an "adrenal androgen synthesis inhibitor." This drug suppresses adrenal androgen production by inhibiting specific enzymes (17-alpha hydroxylase and C17, 20-lyase) that make these androgens. Therefore, it targets the adrenal or androgen pathway more specifically as compared to ketoconazole, so side effects are expected to be less severe and the need for steroid replacement therapy less likely with this drug.

Interestingly, this drug is also believed to work by not allowing the tumor itself to make male hormones, which is why this drug is also known as a "De novo androgen synthesis inhibitor." Tumors have actually figured out a way to make their own testosterone to feed themselves when there is very little or no testosterone available, but abiraterone also seems to work by blocking this unique hormone-producing pathway.

In the ongoing clinical trials, men are *not* allowed to have been on ketoconazole if they want to have the chance of taking abiraterone. However, still-preliminary research has suggested that some men who took ketoconazole also responded to this drug. Another interesting note is that this drug really is an irreversible inhibitor of Cytochrome P450 CYP17A1, which is an enzyme system involved in controlling androgen synthesis from cholesterol precursors. This basically means that it can reduce testosterone to undetectable levels.

Doses from 250 mg to 2000 mg have been studied. For example, in phase-2 studies, 1000 mg daily for 28-day cycles or in combination with prednisone (5 mg) was a popular safe and effective choice.

Side effects will still be a slight concern with this drug because the enzymes that are blocked by the drug lead to an increase in production of a compound called deoxycorticosterone (also known as a "mineralcorticoid"), which can increase blood pressure. Therefore, hypertension is a potential side effect of the drug. Secondary mineralocorticoid excess, which can cause hypertension, low potassium levels, and lower-limb swelling (edema), can occur, so doctors often prescribe another drug to reduce side effects.

Patients should not take any hormonal dietary supplements such as DHEA while on this medication because it could potentially reduce the efficacy of this drug. DHEA is normally turned into androstendione and then into testosterone. Abiraterone blocks DHEA from also being produced, so taking DHEA supplies the tumor with exactly the thing the drug is not allowing the tumor to use to help itself grow.

It is safe to say that patients will continue to hear more about Jevtana and Abiraterone in the future.

Notes

Other Considerations

Exciting Treatments *in the* Immediate *Pipeline*

Chapter Eight

A drug that is in a phase-3 clinical trial has the potential to be approved soon, several years in the future, or perhaps not at all. By checking with your doctor or visiting www.clinicaltrials.gov, you can get the latest information on the status of any drug. For our purposes here in this chapter, we're considering only phase-3 drugs, as those in phase 1 or phase 2 may still be many years from FDA approval.

We have noted whether the drug is available for the "Compassionate Use" or "Expanded Access" program. Check with your health care professional or the drug's company to determine if this is a possibility for your condition. Remember to always check if you are interested as the status on drugs may change from day to day. Be sure to check on insurance coverage and out-of-pocket costs, too.

Drugs to Watch Now

ABIRATERONE ACETATE

Also known as Abiraterone

How is it taken? pill

Approval status one successful phase-3 trial completed and one ongoing

Company Johnson & Johnson

Compassionate use available: yes

Possible advantages This drug was mentioned in chapter seven following the successful completion of one phase-3 trial. It is mentioned here because a second phase-3 clinical trial is testing this pill for men with HRPC who have not yet received chemotherapy and are asymptomatic or have mild symptoms. TAK-700 (Company: Millennium and Takeda) is another pill that works somewhat similar to abiraterone. It is being tested before and after chemotherapy in phase-3 trials. Please see chapter seven for more information on Abiraterone.

AFLIBERCEPT

Also known as AVE0005, VEGF Trap

How is it taken? injection or IV

Approval status phase-3 trial
Company Regeneron and Sanofi-Aventis
Compassionate use available: no
Possible advantages This drug is easy to administer. It works by blocking blood vessel growth (anti-angiogenesis inhibitor) so that the tumor cannot feed itself. It is being tested with Taxotere chemotherapy to determine whether it works better than taking Taxotere alone.
The possible catch Not yet available. No compassionate-use program has been established as of this time, so patients are not able to get the drug unless they are in clinical trials. Protein in the urine (kidney changes), hypertension, and hoarseness are some of the side effects observed with this drug, as with other drugs that work in a similar way. In addition, fatigue and injection site reactions are also common side effects of this drug. However, the severity of these side effects has been minimal for most patients in the clinical trials.
What else do I need to know? The drug works by binding and inhibiting a compound known as VEGF (which stimulates some tumors to grow). This is somewhat similar to how the drug bevacizumab works (known as Avastin, used for breast, colon, and lung cancer). However, bevacizumab did not work well in a recent phase-3 clinical trial of patients with HRPC and it had significant side effects. This does not necessarily mean that afliberecept will not work, because it also has some unique features and it can bind and inactivate VEGF at a rate hundreds of times greater than bevacizumab. In other words, aflibercept has greater and broader binding ability than some of the previous drugs in this class that failed recently, so this is why there should be some optimism with this drug. Each dose of the drug has a half-life of 18 days, which is longer as compared to previous drugs, but regular administration will probably be needed.

ATRASENTAN

Also known as Xinlay
How is it taken? pill
Approval status phase-3 trial

Company Abbott
Compassionate use available: no
Possible advantages It is a daily pill with a low rate of side effects, and it may be usable with chemotherapy.
The possible catch Not yet available. No compassionate-use program has been established as of this time, so patients are not able to get it unless they are in clinical trials. It is being tested to determine whether it makes Taxotere chemotherapy work better than Taxotere by itself in men with bone metastasis and HRPC. A previous clinical trial of atrasentan was not successful, so this is potentially the final phase-3 clinical trial that will determine the future of the drug.
What else do I need to know? This drug is known as an endothelin-a receptor antagonist. The only other drug that works in a similar fashion and is currently in phase-3 clinical trials is zibotentan (see later in this chapter). Atrasentan may work by inhibiting cell proliferation, blood vessel growth, and bone remodeling, and simply by reducing blood flow to the tumor. It may also reduce bone pain. Side effects are due the blood-vessel dilation behavior of this class of medications on normal human tissues, and they include edema, nasal allergy–like symptoms, and headache. There were some rare cases of blood pressure reductions (hypotension), low blood levels of sodium (hyponatremia), and heart failure.

DASATINIB

Also known as Sprycel
How is it taken? pill
Approval status phase-3 trial, is FDA approved for some leukemias so it could be used off-label
Company Bristol-Myers-Squibb
Compassionate use available no
Possible advantages This drug has already been approved by the FDA to treat a chronic myelogenous leukemia (CML) that no longer responds to the drug imatinib (Gleevac) and it is also approved to treat acute lymphoblastic leukemia (ALL). Thus oncologists have good experience with this drug, and it could be

given off-label now to some patients. A randomized phase-3 trial of Taxotere with and without dasatinib is being conducted right now. Dasatinib seems to have direct anti-tumor effects, similar to those it displays in patients with leukemia. It may also have some positive impacts on bone health, and these are also being studied in the phase-3 trial. Once-a-day dosing is the regimen being used in the clinical trial, similar to what is used for leukemia.

The possible catch The drug is in phase-3 clinical trials right now, so it is not yet widely available. Researchers are not certain yet whether this drug helps patients with HRPC. Patients are able to get the medication if they are in clinical trials or receive the drug off-label from their doctors. In past studies, dasatinib has caused low blood counts (neutropenia, thrombocytopenia, and anemia), fluid retention (edema), diarrhea, and, in very rare cases, changes in heart rhythm.

What else do I need to know? The drug recently showed potential effectiveness as a first-line treatment for some patients with CML, which means it is a very powerful drug for some types of leukemia. Whether or not this will translate into an impact on HRPC remains to be seen, but at least the drug is available currently for other indications. Other oral drugs that are somewhat similar to this drug have not worked well for HRPC.

IPILIMUMAB

Also known as MDX-010

How is it taken? IV

Approval status phase-3 trial

Company Bristol-Myers-Squibb

Compassionate use available no

Possible advantages The drug is being tested in a variety of prostate cancer situations and stages, including in some smaller studies of men who are also receiving androgen deprivation therapy (ADT) for locally advanced prostate cancer, as well as those getting chemotherapy. The larger phase-3 trial involves men with HRPC who no longer respond to Taxotere chemotherapy. The drug recently showed some success in melanoma patients, so off-label opportunities may open up for men with more limited options. It has a unique mechanism of action: allowing the body to maximize its own immune response.

The possible catch No compassionate-use program has been established as of this time, so patients are not able to get it unless they are in a clinical trial (this could change if the drug becomes available off-label because it gets approved for another kind of cancer, such as melanoma). The potential for an overactive immune response to cause numerous side effects also needs to be further understood. Is it possible that this drug could create some serious autoimmune condition, so that the immune system also attacks healthy cells of the body, such as the liver? It is possible, and this has happened. The phase-3 trial will provide much more clarity for the side-effect issues, and some patients may be treated with steroid medications if serious toxicity occurs.

What else do I need to know? Ipilimumab is an immune system–activating drug that is actually a human antibody. It binds and blocks a site on specific immune cells (T cells) known as CTLA4 (Cytotoxic T Lymphocyte–associated Antigen 4) to improve the body's immune response to a cancer. Thus far, it has received the most clinical research with melanoma or skin cancer. Why do immune cells even need CTLA4? CTLA4 is normally needed to help keep the immune system in balance so it will not overreact to certain situations and attack healthy cells. However, cancer cells help to keep the immune system from being activated, causing the need for this drug. The excitement around this drug really centers on the fact that if it indeed helps to fight melanoma, one of the most aggressive types of cancer, then the possibility that it may have an impact on many other cancers seems more likely.

LENALIDOMIDE

Also known as Revlimid

How is it taken? pill

Approval status phase-3 trial, FDA-approved for another cancer so can be used off-label

Company Celgene

Compassionate use available no

Possible advantages This drug is known for having multiple effects, such as blocking blood vessel tumor growth, immune enhancement, and anti-inflammatory effects. The drug is approved right now for multiple myeloma, so there is a chance that some men with HRPC could get this drug off-label.

The possible catch No compassionate use program has been established as of this time, so patients are not able to get the drug unless they are in a clinical trial or from possible off-label use. A range of side effects has occurred, from gastrointestinal problems to fatigue to blood cell reductions and blood clots, in patients using this drug for other conditions, so be sure to review these with your doctor.

What else do I need to know? This drug is being tested in combination with Taxotere chemotherapy to determine whether it works better than Taxotere alone for men with metastatic HRPC. Since this drug has been approved in another area of cancer treatment, there is optimism that it may increase the effectiveness of chemotherapy for prostate cancer. The drug is somewhat similar to the drug thalidomide, which is notoriously known for its toxicity when taken decades ago by pregnant women, but lenalidomide may be advantageous in treating some types of cancer patients because of its multiple mechanisms of action.

MDV3100

How is it taken? pill

Approval status multiple phase-3 trials

Company Medivation Inc.

Compassionate use available no

Possible advantages This is a pill with a low rate of side effects, and it is one of the most potent anti-androgen drugs ever invented. It seems to also encourage prostate cancer cell death. This drug does not require that a steroid drug be taken with it, so combining it with immune therapies is an exciting possibility.

The possible catch Not available yet unless you enroll in a clinical trial, and there is no compassionate use currently available.

One clinical trial will test daily MDV3100 by itself against a placebo in men who are no longer responding to Taxotere. The primary side effect of this drug in clinical trials has been dose-dependent fatigue. It has taken about 4 weeks to occur in some patients, which is about the time it takes the drug to reach higher concentrations in the body. A small percentage of patients have also reported nausea and weight loss.

What else do I need to know? Androgen receptors are actually increased in HRPC. If a drug could tightly bind to the androgen receptor, it would make it difficult for anything else to fit into that receptor and stimulate tumor growth. Anti-androgen pills available on the market today, such as bicalutamide, flutamide, and nilutamide, are not able to bind as tightly to the androgen receptor as MDV3100. Theoretically, this pill could work to reduce tumor growth in HRPC. Patients who have responded to this drug in past clinical trials are the ones who have stopped responding to other anti-androgens, demonstrating the effectiveness of MDV3100.

OGX-011

Also known as custirsen sodium

How is it taken? IV

Approval status phase-3 trial

Company OncoGenex

Compassionate use available no

Possible advantages It is an intravenous (IV) drug given at regular intervals (about once a week). The drug stays in the body for a long time, so it may not have to be given very frequently. Regular doses of chemotherapy may possibly be given with it. Several phase-2 clinical studies have demonstrated that this drug seems to work best with Taxotere.

The possible catch The drug is in phase-3 clinical trials right now, so it is not yet available. No compassionate-use program has been established as of this time, so patients are not able to get it unless they are in clinical trials. Side effects in previous studies include chills (involuntary muscle contractions), fever, and increased blood levels of creatinine (kidney changes).

What else do I need to know? The drug looks promising in combination with Taxotere chemotherapy, which is why a phase-3 study of men with HRPC has been initiated. The drug is able to reduce or block the production of a compound, clusterin, that is over expressed in HRPC. Clusterin seems to help tumors survive and helps to create drug resistance. Blood levels of clusterin can be measured in clinical trials, and the large reduction in these blood levels may correlate with a treatment response. The ability of this drug to also reduce pain is being studied in men with HRPC. The drug is currently being studied in breast cancer and advanced non–small cell lung cancer.

PROSTVAC

Also known as poxviral vaccine
How is it taken? injection
Approval status phase-3 trial
Company Bavarian Nordic
Compassionate use available no
Possible advantages This vaccine uses 2 weakened pox viruses that have been genetically altered to produce slightly abnormal versions of PSA, and also has 3 molecules that may boost the immune system. Officially it is called a "poxviral prostate-specific antigen (PSA) targeted recombinant viral vaccine." Researchers completed a phase-2 clinical trial of 125 men at 43 centers in the United States. Median survival was 25.1 months for those who received the vaccine and 16.6 months in the placebo group (an 8.5 month difference). This was equivalent to a 44 percent reduction in the rate of death.
The possible catch The drug is in phase-3 clinical trials now, so it is not yet available. No compassionate-use program has been established as of this time, so patients are not able to get it unless they are in clinical trials. Side effects in previous studies include a small number of injection site reactions and fatigue, fever, and nausea.
What else do I need to know? Studies need to be completed to determine the effectiveness of this vaccine. One consideration is that men in the placebo group were older and had higher median PSA levels. Almost 10 percent of men in the

vaccine group had lymph node–only positive disease, compared to none in the vaccine group, and more patients in the vaccine group had disease in the bones only. It is possible that the men in the vaccine group had a slightly better prognosis, or it is possible that this vaccine may be working very well and that these slight differences in clinical characteristics did not really matter in the results. This is why a final phase-3 trial is needed. It is interesting that the progression of the disease in this situation (known as progression-free survival or PFS) and PSA level was generally not impacted when it was measured at 6 months. This continues to suggest that these immune-boosting therapies work in a special way to help patients live longer and that researchers have not been able to figure out how and why precisely just yet.

RADIUM-223

Also known as Alpharadin
How is it taken? IV
Approval status phase-3 trial
Company Algeta
Compassionate use available no
Possible advantages This is a radiopharmaceutical drug (radioactive IV drug) that will be given every 4 weeks for a total of 6 cycles for men with bone metastasis and symptomatic HRPC who are not candidates for Taxotere chemotherapy, in order to determine whether it can improve survival. This drug and others somewhat similar to it (samarium and strontium, both already approved for metastatic HRPC) reduce pain by going into the body, seeking cancerous areas, and emitting energy particles that kill cancer cells so that individuals get some pain relief rather quickly (usually within a week).
The possible catch No compassionate-use program has been established as of this time, so patients are not able to get it unless they are in a clinical trial. The side effects from this drug result from radiation that goes into the bone and can cause blood cell production (white blood cells and platelets) to be reduced. Less commonly, diarrhea can occur.

What else do I need to know? Radium emits alpha radiation, which means it contains more radiation that travels a shorter distance as compared to other radiopharmaceutical drugs in this class, so the benefit-to-risk ratio may be better for patients. All of the radiopharmaceutical drugs work well for bone pain and are probably underused in HRPC patients.

XL184

Also known as Cabozantinib
How is it taken? pill
Approval status phase 3 trial begins soon
Company Exelixis
Compassionate use available no
Possible advantages This is a pill (may also come in a liquid form) that is given daily. It is moving quickly toward a phase-3 trial now. The phase-2 results in HRPC showed that this drug reduced or stabilized metastatic bone lesions in nearly all patients who were evaluated by a bone scan. The drug also reduced bone pain and the need for narcotic pain medication, and increased hemoglobin levels in patients with anemia. It may also shrink tumors in some organs of the body (liver, lungs, etc.).
The possible catch The median time patients were followed in the phase-2 study thus far is only several months (some were followed for less than 1 month and others for more than 1 year), so researchers are not sure if patients will also do better in the long-term. Fatigue, reduced appetite, other gastrointestinal issues, and an increase in blood pressure were some of the side effects that were increased with this drug in some patients. However, the percentage of patients who experienced serious problems with these side effects or other serious side effects was very low. For example, extreme fatigue requiring more clinical attention occurred in only 15 percent of patients, and a serious reduction in appetite occurred in 2 percent of patients.
What else do I need to know? XL184 is a small molecule that was designed to block signals allowing a tumor to grow. It is a compound that disrupts the ability of a tumor to feed itself and probably works in multiple other ways to stop the signals that allow

a tumor to grow. This drug is also being studied in patients with certain types of thyroid cancer, brain tumors, lung cancer, and other cancers that have advanced, such as pancreatic, liver, gastric, melanoma, breast, and ovarian cancer. In fact, the drug is in the final phase-3 trial for patients with medullary thyroid cancer.

ZIBOTENTAN

Also known as ZD4054
How is it taken? pill
Approval status phase-3 trial
Company AstraZeneca
Compassionate use available no
Possible advantages This is a pill given daily. It is in phase-3 clinical trials right now. The medication is simple to take and has minimal side effects. It is somewhat similar to the drug atrasentan (see earlier).
The possible catch The drug is in phase-3 clinical trials right now, so it is not yet available. No compassionate-use program has been established as of this time, so that patients are not able to get it unless they are in clinical trials. Edema (fluid retention), headaches, and nasal congestion are some of the more frequent side effects (similar to the drug atrasentan mentioned earlier). It was already tested in a phase-3 trial of non-metastatic HRPC patients. The drug did not demonstrate a positive effect in the study.
What else do I need to know? This drug belongs in a category of endothelin receptor antagonists, and it is being used in clinical trials as a single agent or in combination with chemotherapy.

As you can see, this is definitely an exciting period in HRPC research, with many promising treatments in phase-3 testing. In the appendix at the back of the book, you'll find a listing of some of the phase-1 and phase-2 drugs being studied, as well as some of the off-label drugs that physicians consider for HRPC treatment. Chapter nine will provide tips on preventing and lessening side effects of the many treatments we've considered to this point.

Preventing *and* Lessening *Side* Effects

Chapter Nine

Side effects to be covered in this chapter:

- Acid Reflux
- Allergic Reactions
- Anemia
- Bone Loss
- Breast Pain and Enlargement
- Breathing Difficulty
- Cholesterol Level Changes
- Cognitive Impairment
- Constipation
- Depression and Mood Changes
- Diarrhea
- Dry Skin and Dermatitis
- Erectile Dysfunction and Loss of Libido
- Fatigue
- Fever
- Fluid Retention
- Hair Loss
- Hot Flashes
- Incontinence
- Insomnia
- Joint Pain
- Mouth and Canker Sores
- Muscle Loss and Pain
- Nail Changes
- Nausea and Vomiting
- Neuropathy
- Neutropenia
- Nosebleeds
- Pain
- Penis and Scrotum Shrinkage
- Stress and Anxiety
- Sweating
- Taste Changes
- Testosterone Deficiency Syndrome
- Thrombocytopenia
- Tingling and Numbness
- Watery Eyes
- Weight Gain
- Weight Loss

For patients considering various treatments for HRPC, side effects are an important part of the equation. Not only will they impact the patient's quality of life, but they may also result in a necessity to delay, reduce, or terminate a treatment program. It is always important to ask your doctor about the common and rarer side effects of any treatment before starting it to help you evaluate your options. Fortunately, there are many ways to both prevent and alleviate many of the undesirable effects of cancer treatment. In this chapter, we'll give suggestions for lifestyle and diet tips, supplements and over-the-counter treatments, and prescription medications that work on each side effect. You should be candid in discussing your symptoms with your doctor to find the best solutions for your situation.

Side effects are usually graded in clinical trials using a scale that is easy to understand.

Following is one of the most popular side effect grading systems:

1 = mild
2 = moderate
3 = severe
4 = life threatening or disabling
5 = fatal

Grade 1 and 2 side effects are generally preventable and treatable, and often do not last for a long time. A drug that has many grade 1 and 2 side effects and very few grade 3 or 4 side effects is usually considered a safe drug.

Please keep in mind that grade 3 or 4 side effects are usually reported separately from overall side effects in clinical trials because these are the side effects that interfere with your "activities of daily living" (ADL). It is always important when talking about new treatments to determine the *percentage* of patients who had grade 3 or 4 side effects and what *specific* side effects in the study were grade 3 or 4. Also consider the potential preventive and treatment options for any of the side effects (grades 1 to 4). Since grade 5 side effects caused death, they are also important to consider, although they are very rare generally.

ACID REFLUX

Also known as heartburn, indigestion, gastric reflux, gastroesophageal reflux disease, or GERD

What is it? Why does it happen? Acid reflux occurs when some of the acidic stomach contents move into the esophagus, the pipe that carries food from the mouth to the stomach. It can occur due to weight gain or lifestyle choices. It can run in families or be caused by some medications. Medications that increase the risk of acid reflux include antacids that are used for too long (the body develops rebound acid reflux), antibiotics, some antidepressants, some cancer treatments, over-the-counter and prescription pain medications, and even steroid medications such as prednisone. Over time, the acidic contents of the stomach can irritate and also slightly burn into the esophageal lining and cause numerous problems.

What are the signs or symptoms? Symptoms include a burning sensation in your chest, a taste of sour liquid or regurgitated food in the back of your mouth, frequent heartburn, indigestion, and trouble swallowing. In some instances, individuals do not realize they are experiencing acid reflux because their symptoms are less typical, but keep in mind that a chronic cough, wheezing, and even mild chest pain especially while lying down at night can also be due to this problem.

Note *It is important to keep in mind that some of the medications used to treat heartburn, particularly prescription treatments and newer over-the-counter drugs, can be so effective at reducing stomach acid that they may in rare circumstances also reduce the absorption of some drugs. One drug of particular concern in conjunction with antacids is ketoconazole. However, there are a number of options, discussed below, that may work without causing that concern.*

Prevention and Treatment Options

Lifestyle and Diet Tips

- Eliminate any tobacco products and reduce caffeine and alcohol. All of these substances contribute to acid reflux.
- Some physicians recommend reducing chocolate consumption. Research on this has been mixed, so monitor chocolate intake to see if it bothers your digestive system.
- Losing just a little bit of weight takes some pressure off the stomach and can immediately reduce reflux.

- Sleeping with your head elevated or on your left side helps keep stomach acid down in the stomach.
- Eating smaller meals avoids overfilling the stomach. Particularly watch large meals at dinner or near bedtime.
- Eliminating fried or fatty foods, or beverages or pills that are acidic (citrus fruit juices, alcoholic beverages, and plain vitamin C tablets) and not required by your doctor. They can make your condition worse. Look for non-acidic options or alternatives. For example, calcium ascorbate or buffered vitamin C is not as harsh on the stomach as plain vitamin C.
- Fiber is your best friend here. Flaxseed, chia seed, oatmeal, bran cereals, or even fiber powder supplements in small amounts all work like a sponge to mop up acid. Try to get 25 to 30 grams of fiber per day. It is one of the only things in your diet that clinical research has found to be consistent at reducing acid reflux. You'll find a list of high-fiber foods in the section on constipation.
- Try not to exercise on a full stomach

Dietary Supplements and Over-the-Counter Options

- There are many over-the-counter (OTC) antacids, including calcium carbonate and aluminum or magnesium hydroxide (Rolaids, Tums, Maalox, and Mylanta). There are also numerous prescription drugs that are now offered in an over-the-counter strength, including famotidine (Pepcid) and ranitidine (Zantac), Prevacid and Prilosec, together with many generic pharmacy competitors. These OTC options now come in many delivery options, such as liquid, chews, and tablets.
- If you do go on any acid-reducing OTC or prescription drug long term, you may have a calcium absorption problem. Calcium citrate is absorbed well, either with or without food, and also in a low-acid stomach. This is not always the case with the other calcium supplements.
- Enzyme-based dietary supplements help to reduce gas in

the digestive tract, which may result from reflux disease or excessive stomach acid produced in the digestion process of some foods. One of the most popular is the enzyme alpha-galactosidase (Beano). It actually comes from a fungus (Aspergillus), and it breaks down sugars found in some foods, such as beans and vegetables, so that they cannot cause bloating and gas. Other products on the market contain simethicone (Gas-X, for one), which is an anti-foaming agent. In addition, peppermint oil supplements, ginger, and even chamomile all work as stomach muscle relaxants and can help to reduce gas. Keep in mind that excess gas is caused by many things, but it does occur in some individuals with acid reflux and that these supplements may help.

- Deglycyrrhizinated licorice (DGL) is a dietary supplement promoted in many alternative medicine books for ulcers, heartburn, acid reflux, and all kinds of gastrointestinal disorders. This herb should *not* be used by cancer patients because it has the potential to interact negatively with steroid medication and cause blood pressure swings. Please stay away from this supplement until clinical research shows that it is safe during HRPC treatment.

Prevention and Treatment Options

The most effective products are either the H2 blockers or the even more popular proton-pump inhibitors (PPIs). Some effective medications are:

- Aciphex (rabeprazole)
- Nexium (esomeprazole)
- Prevacid (lansoprazole, also over the counter now)
- Prilosec (omeprazole, also over the counter now)
- Protonix (pantoprazole)
- Zantac (ranitidine)

As mentioned, there is a slight catch with taking the acid reflux drugs over the long term: they can reduce the absorption of calcium, and they reduce the efficacy of the second-line hormone drug ketoconazole. Also, these drugs may slightly increase the risk of certain gastrointestinal infections and pneumonia because they are so effective at reducing stomach acid. When stomach acid is reduced, this also reduces an important immune barrier that normally eliminates any bad microorganisms that hit the stomach. However, this overall risk is very small.

There are other drugs that work in different ways to provide relief. For example, promotility agents help to empty the stomach. A couple of these drugs are metoclopramide (Reglan) and bethanechol.

There is also a coating-agent drug called sucralfate (Carafate) that helps to provide a coating to sensitive areas so that stomach acid cannot erode the surrounding tissue.

Lastly, there are various medical procedures that can be discussed with your doctor for severe acid reflux that lifestyle changes and medication cannot solve. However, such options are needed only in rare cases today.

ALLERGIC REACTIONS

Also known as hypersensitivity reactions

What is it? Why does it happen? When receiving any new drug it is always possible, but thankfully rare, that a person experiences a mild, moderate, or even severe allergic reaction to it. Some individuals may be sensitive to any new medication, or may even develop an allergic reaction to a medication over time. Medication allergies are similar to allergies in general, in that some people have a lot of them and some have none at all. Some allergies go away with time, and some get worse with time. While it is possible to experience a reaction to most, if not all, medications, some are definitely more likely to create allergic reactions, such as penicillin.

Additionally, when receiving any infusion of any drug, the human body may simply develop an allergic reaction to the infusion itself because the process of infusion does introduce a non-familiar material to the skin and body. It is not unusual for some health-care professionals to develop an allergy to certain materials, such as latex, that can be found in some surgical gloves.

The good news is that it is rare to have an allergic reaction to any medication, and physicians have several preventive allergy therapies that are used in cancer treatment and plenty of ways to treat an allergic reaction. Thankfully, it is extremely rare to have a serious allergic reaction to a cancer drug that could require hospitalization or that is life-threatening.

What are the signs or symptoms? In general, allergic reactions tend to occur most often within the first few minutes of taking a drug or getting an infusion. However, in some cases, it can also occur anytime during an infusion. Mild-to-moderate allergic reactions usually involve one or more of the following symptoms: itching, flushing, rash (with or without itching), difficulty breathing or chest tightness, back pain, fever, chills, and low blood pressure.

Severe allergic reactions include: serious difficulty breathing, severe drops in blood pressure, and extensive itching and rash throughout the body. A mild-to-moderate allergic reaction still may permit treatment with a cancer drug if the drug is tried at a slower rate or introduced into the body in a smaller amount over time to limit the reaction. However, in rare cases where the allergic reaction to the drug is severe, the offending drug is completely stopped, and a substitute drug or another therapy is recommended.

Prevention and Treatment Options

Lifestyle and Diet Tips

One of the most important things that you can do to prevent allergic reactions is to clearly identify to your doctor any previous allergies to medication that you believe you have had, and indicate what specifically happened during that allergic reaction (itching, fainting, blood pressure changes, rash, flushing, bumps on skin, etc.). This will allow health care professionals to accurately document the allergies in your medical record.

Always pay attention to any strange feelings, especially during the early minutes of any infusion, because this is when most allergic reactions occur. Things to watch for include: itching, redness, bumps, breathing changes, flushing, and slightly elevated swellings of the skin. A health worker usually waits in the room during the first few minutes after the start of any infusion with important anti-allergy medical interventions (antihistamines, steroids, epinephrine, bronchodilators, and an oxygen supply), and blood pressure is usually monitored for some cancer treatments.

It is important to realize that most advanced cancer drugs have not been clinically tested for allergic reactions when combined with other drugs. Since many cancer drugs are metabolized through the same part of the liver and intestines as foods, be careful about choosing foods or beverages that could theoretically block drug metabolism and cause higher-than-normal blood levels of certain drugs. For example, grapefruit, grapefruit juice, and other items (such as Seville oranges) could cause these reactions. Check with a pharmacist or your doctor for the latest list of foods and beverages that can change the metabolism of your cancer drug.

Individuals may also experience a minor allergic reaction to alcohol use or overuse. Alcohol can actually contain histamine or cause a histamine release and allergy-like symptoms in many individuals. Beer (from the wheat and other compounds), wine (with preservatives such as sulfites), and even hard liquor have all been known to elicit an allergy-type reaction, so drink in moderation or not at all.

Dietary Supplements and Over-the-Counter Options

While undergoing cancer treatment, please do not add any new herbal products or dietary supplements to your regimen without talking to your doctor first. This is especially true around the time you are to receive an infusion of any drug or any new cancer medication. Many dietary supplements can increase or decrease the metabolism of your cancer drug, and there are many dietary supplements that have no impact on your cancer drug. However, it is always better to be safe rather than sorry and not combine any new supplement with any new drug.

Fish oil or omega-3 and vitamin D are commonly touted to

have the ability to reduce allergic reactions, but this is really not true. In fact, some people have allergies to fish and fish oil, and it can also cause blood thinning. No good research shows that vitamin D prevents allergies, so never take either of these supplements to prevent or treat a drug allergy.

Proven over-the-counter medications to reduce or treat allergies include diphenhydramine (Benadryl) and antihistamine drugs (such as loratadine or cetirizine). These will usually be provided by your doctor's office if you need them before an infusion is given. If you purchase these medications ahead of time, you should note that they all come in less-expensive generic options that contain exactly the same ingredients. It is a good idea to purchase diphenhydramine in whichever form you prefer—liquid, tablets, melts, or stripes—and leave one box in your house and travel with another. This medication can help anyone who is having an allergic reaction away from the clinic. They are good to use in an emergency until medical attention can be obtained for a medication or food allergy, or even a bee sting.

Although over-the-counter hydrocortisone cream can treat some skin allergic reactions, this is rarely needed in cancer treatment because there are far more powerful medications that can treat an allergic reaction. However, sometimes acetaminophen (Tylenol) or a pain medication is also given during an infusion to reduce any discomfort associated with the process (pain at the infusion site, general discomfort, or aches and pains after the infusion).

Prescriptions and Medical Procedures

If there is any concern regarding an allergic reaction with a cancer drug, your doctor will also prescribe a steroid pill (for example prednisone), which can be taken regularly to prevent or minimize any problems. Giving a "test" dosage of a drug to determine allergic potential has been discussed, but when tested using Taxotere chemotherapy, for example, this process was not generally effective in reducing the severity of a future allergic reactions. Therefore, receiving a steroid medication from the doctor seems the best course to reduce the small risk of allergies.

Additionally, an IV form of diphenhydramine (Benadryl) or IV steroids (dexamethasone, for one) can be given at the time the allergy occurs, such as at infusion time.

Epinephrine injections or EPI pens are given to some patients who have very serious or even life-threatening reactions to certain foods (peanuts, for example), medications, or even bee stings. When the serious allergy develops, patients are taught to plunge the pen or needle in the outer thigh (not toward the inside thigh or the buttocks) and to hold the device in place for about 10 seconds to deliver the life-saving medication. Although these EPI pens are rarely given to cancer patients, some cancer patients have to carry them because of other allergies. Always carry your EPI pen with you if your doctor prescribes one.

Bronchodilators open up constricting air passages during an allergic reaction and are sometimes prescribed to patients.

In summary, antihistamines, steroids, epinephrine, and bronchodilators (even an oxygen supply) are just some of the many medical interventions that can alleviate an allergic reaction.

ANEMIA

Also known as low blood cell count

What is it? Why does it occur? Blood, more specifically red blood cells, is less able to carry oxygen to supply energy to cells throughout the body due either to a decrease in number of cells or a problem with the cells themselves.

Anemia usually happens with androgen deprivation therapy (ADT), and it occurs in the first few months of treatment in 90 percent of men. Testosterone is used in producing a hormone that helps maintain a normal red blood cell count, so a large reduction in testosterone is a common cause of this problem in patients having ADT. The type of anemia that usually occurs with ADT is known as a "normochromic normocytic" anemia, which simply means that the body is still producing normal red blood cells, just not enough of them.

As was discussed earlier, it is also common for chemotherapy to have an effect on bone marrow and on the production of blood cells. Chemotherapy is designed to have a toxic effect on rapidly dividing tumor cells, and unfortunately it is often also toxic to healthy rapidly dividing cells such as the ones in bone marrow that produce red and white blood cells. In fact, anemia is one of the more common possible side effects of chemotherapy.

What are the signs or symptoms? The symptoms a person experiences will depend on the severity of the anemia. They can range from no symptoms in mild cases to include some of the ones below in more severe cases:

- Fatigue
- Dizziness or feeling faint
- Shortness of breath
- Feeling as if your heart is pounding
- Pale skin
- Chest pain
- Numbness or coldness in hands and feet
- Headaches

Your doctor may run lab tests from time to time to check to be sure that your blood cell counts are normal.

Prevention and Treatment Options

Most men do not need treatment for this condition when it is related to ADT treatment, because the reduction in red blood cell count is usually only 10 percent. After several months, it either resolves itself or simply does not cause symptoms.

Lifestyle and Diet Tips

If your doctor feels that it is advisable for your condition, weightlifting or resistance exercise can help to reduce the risk of this condition. A study from Australia showed that lifting weights just two to three times a week may help to stimulate red blood cell production in men on ADT. Doctors do not usually want to give testosterone or another medication to improve this condition unless it is really needed.

If you experience fatigue from the anemia, please check out some of the suggestions in the upcoming fatigue section. Drink plenty of fluids as this will help keep you from feeling dizzy when you stand or sit up. If you do feel light-headed, be sure to stand up slowly if you are sitting or lying down.

Dietary Supplements and Over-the-Counter Options

None recommended.

Prescriptions and Medical Procedures

Effective prescription medications, such as recombinant erythropoietin (Epogen, Aranesp, or Procrit) that will help produce more red blood cells are always available if the anemia is severe. Additionally, a blood transfusion is an option in some situations.

BONE LOSS

Also known as osteoporosis

What is it? Why does it happen? Osteoporosis is a weakening of your bones that can lead to an increased risk of bone fracture. Any treatment that affects or simply reduces male hormone levels (ADT) may cause bone loss or weakness. Since most men being treated for HRPC receive ADT at some point, this side effect merits some consideration.

Additionally, as was discussed earlier in the book, a high percentage of prostate cancer recurrences involve the bones. Patients with HRPC can be vulnerable to skeletal-related events (SREs), including fractures, spinal cord compression, and hypercalcemia (bones that release dangerous amounts of calcium into the blood). These SREs negatively affect the quality of life for patients and provide another reason to focus on improving bone strength. Please review the use of Zometa and Xgeva to treat SREs in chapter three. We'll discuss it briefly later in this section as well.

What are the signs or symptoms? Tell your doctor about any pain you feel, even if you think it might be due to some other problem, such as arthritis or stiffness from lack of activity or a muscle pull or strain. Often there are no symptoms of bone loss until a bone fracture occurs, so we need to consider how to prevent this from happening. First, we will discuss how bone loss is diagnosed.

An imaging (picture) test is used to help determine the status of your bone health. An imaging test usually takes a picture of one or several sites of the body. Then your bones are compared to those of a 25- to 30-year-old male, the benchmark age range where individuals have optimal bone health. If your bone or bones are similar to the benchmark, then this is considered normal. If your bones are a little less dense or a little weaker than the benchmark, this is called osteopenia. Osteoporosis occurs when your bones are much weaker than the benchmark. Finally, if you have already had a fracture and your bones are much weaker than a young person's, this is called severe osteoporosis. The weaker your bones are compared to a young person's, and the more bone loss you have experienced, the more likely it is that you will experience a fracture in the future unless intervention occurs that reduces your risk of continued bone loss.

There are several devices available today to help your doctor determine the relative state of your bones. The two most common are compared in the following chart. At some point in your cancer treatment, your doctor may suggest that you have one of these tests.

Test	**Dual-Energy X-ray Absorptiometry (DEXA)**
Advantages	Fairly inexpensive. Low radiation exposure. Rapid and easy to perform. Most multiple site-specific test for spine, hip, wrist. Recommended for most men.
Limitations	Osteoarthritis of the lumbar spine and/or aortic calcifications falsely elevate measurement in older patients.
Test	**Quantitative Computerized Tomography (QCT)**
Advantages	Most sensitive method to detect osteoporosis of the spine. Recommended for some men when DEXA is not adequate.
Limitations	Expensive. High-dose radiation exposure for patient.

Lifestyle and Diet Tips

CALCIUM CONTENT PER SERVING	
Collard greens	360 mg
Orange juice (fortified)	350 mg
Sardines	325 mg
Oatmeal (instant)	325 mg
Yogurt	300 mg
Milk	300 mg
Spinach	290 mg
Cheese	270 mg

Weightlifting or resistance exercise and regular aerobic exercise of any type are the best ways to reduce the risk of bone loss and weakness. It is important to check with your doctor to see what exercise program best fits your situation, but, if it is an option for you, exercise improves bone health.

Consuming calcium-rich foods is also a good base for other treatment possibilities. Review the list and pick your favorites.

Dietary Supplements and Over-the-Counter Options

Recent research suggests that most men on ADT do not get the recommended daily intake of calcium, which is 1200 to 1500 mg per day, an amount that, along with vitamin D, may help improve bone strength. Only 1 to 2 pills of a calcium supplement per day should be enough to meet your daily intake.

Recent research with vitamin D suggests that supplementation with an average of 800–1000 IU may help reduce bone loss, but ideally it would be best to first get a vitamin D blood test (25-OH vitamin D test) before deciding with your doctor whether you need more or less.

Prescriptions and Medical Procedures

The most commonly utilized pills or IV medications to prevent bone loss in prostate cancer patients are a class of drugs known as bisphosphonates. They include many different types of prescription pills, such as alendronate (Fosamax), ibandronate (Boniva), and risedronate (Actonel). However, the most commonly used of these medications are Zometa or Xgeva. While all of these drugs will potentially improve bone strength, Zometa is the only FDA approved bisphosphonate that also lowers the incidence of skeletal-related events (SREs) in prostate cancer patients. Xgeva may also be useful in preventing SREs, so please ask your doctor if that is a choice for you.

Research also suggests that a class of drugs known as selective estrogen receptor modulators (SERMs) may prevent bone loss. The most commonly used drugs are raloxifene and toremifene, which are both in clinical trials for men and have to be taken daily. Talk to your doctor about potential side effects (blood clots, etc.) of these medications.

There is some preliminary research showing that some of the osteoporosis drugs (especially Zometa and Xgeva), which work so well to prevent bone loss, may also help to slow the progression of prostate cancer or block the ability of cancer to invade the bone. This is very preliminary. You should ask your doctor about this because these drugs also come with drawbacks and the possibility exists that they may be overprescribed in some cases where just lifestyle changes and dietary supplements could prevent bone loss.

As was mentioned in chapter four, they may increase the risk of serious jawbone issues (such as osteonecrosis of the jaw). If considering these treatments, it is a good idea to first get clearance from a dentist to remove any suspicious areas of potential infection (for example, a partially impacted wisdom tooth). If a man is already taking these drugs, he should continue to see his dentist on a regular basis.

BREAST PAIN AND ENLARGEMENT

Also known as gynecomastia

What is it? Why does it happen? In men undergoing some treatments for prostate cancer, nipples of the breast become sensitive and painful and/or the amount of breast tissue increases. Anti-androgen treatment (bicalutamide, flutamide, and nilutamide) is often responsible for this side effect. The greater the dosage, the greater the chance of it occurring during the course of treatment. Estrogen given to men (as well as rarely dutasteride and finasteride) can also cause this problem.

What are the signs or symptoms? Tenderness or swelling in breast tissue.

Prevention and Treatment Options

Lifestyle and Diet Tips

None.

Dietary Supplements and Over-the-Counter Options

None.

Prescriptions and Medical Procedures

There are two effective ways to prevent gynecomastia. The first is to take a daily anti-estrogen prescription pill, such as tamoxifen or any drug known as an aromatase inhibitor. These work by blocking the ability of estrogen to stimulate the breast tissue in men. The only problem is that this pill usually has to be taken daily.

The other effective preventive method is to receive a small dose of radiation to each breast (prophylactic breast irradiation). This takes very little time and usually only needs to be done one time. Early intervention with either of these methods may improve outcomes.

Finally, for men who have already experienced significant breast enlargement, a specialist can surgically remove some of this tissue, if desired.

BREATHING DIFFICULTY

Also known as dyspnea

This serious side effect can occur for a number of reasons during cancer treatment. Patients are advised to seek medical attention right away if they experience breathing difficulty or any other serious side effect, such as chest pain, dizziness or loss of consciousness, or vision changes. They are potentially life-threatening side effects and, as thus, require immediate medical attention.

CHOLESTEROL LEVEL CHANGES

What is it? Why does it happen? When considering a patient's total cholesterol as measured by a blood test, some prostate cancer treatments tend to increase LDL (bad cholesterol) and/or triglycerides, and decrease HDL (good cholesterol). Anti-androgen pills (bicalutamide, for example) are responsible for lowering HDL when combined with androgen deprivation treatment. Additionally, ADT can increase triglycerides in some men.

However, ADT by itself can also significantly increase HDL. This may come as a surprise to many health-care professionals and patients, but it has been a consistent finding in clinical trials. This actually makes sense, because high amounts of testosterone can lower HDL.

Whether or not ADT impacts the risk of heart disease is not clear, but these findings reinforce the recommendation that prostate cancer patients need to know their cholesterol numbers as well as they know their PSA. This just makes sense in light of the fact that cardiovascular disease is the number-one cause of death in men.

What are the signs or symptoms? None.

Prevention and Treatment Options

Lifestyle and Diet Tips

There are so many wonderful lifestyle changes that can impact your cholesterol in a positive way. Several quick tips can help improve your cholesterol numbers:

- Get rid of a few pounds. If you weigh more than you should, slimming down may provide a significant drop in your cholesterol, especially by reducing triglycerides.
- Regular exercise can increase good cholesterol (HDL).
- Learn the "good fats." Cutting fat from your diet will generally lower cholesterol, but evidence suggests that eating more of some fats and less of others may help with your goal. Monounsaturated fat can help lower LDL and triglycerides, while raising HDL. Omega-3 fatty acids, such as are found in fish, can also be a good choice. Saturated fats, found primarily in animal products such as meats, butter, full-fat milk, and cheese, can increase cholesterol and should be consumed sparingly.
- Fiber has the ability to lower cholesterol, so eat lots of

fiber by making fruits, vegetables, whole grains, and beans a large part of your diet. The fiber will also make you feel fuller and may contribute to weight loss goals. (See more information on fiber in the section on constipation following.)

- Read food labels carefully to help pick products that are lower in calories, low in saturated and other fats, and high in fiber. Be sure to watch sodium content, too, to improve your overall heart health.

Dietary Supplements and Over-the-Counter Options

Niacin is an excellent medication to improve HDL numbers in men who have lower numbers, and fish oil can reduce triglycerides in those with abnormally high numbers. However, keep in mind that all medications have some side effects, for example, hot flashes or liver problems with niacin and potentially a blood-thinning effect with high doses of fish oil. Red-yeast rice extract supplements can lower LDL, but they can also cause liver problems. Talk to your doctor about the range of options available to improve your cholesterol and lower your heart disease risk.

Prescriptions and Medical Procedures

"Statin" or cholesterol-lowering drug treatments have been very successful for men who cannot control their cholesterol through lifestyle changes. In addition, recent evidence suggests that these medications may have an anti-prostate cancer effect. There are numerous studies underway. Even if the drugs do not prove to have that benefit in the end, at least they can reduce the risk of the leading cause of death in men—heart disease.

COGNITIVE IMPAIRMENT

What is it? Why does it happen? Patients can develop the inability to remember some things and/or a feeling of mental fogginess or slowness. Some studies show that ADT or chemotherapy might cause this, but the effect is rare, and other studies have shown no impact with these treatments. Regardless, if there is any concern at all, please talk to your doctor.

What are the signs or symptoms? Patients may notice themselves forgetting things they would normally remember and may feel a bit mentally "fuzzy."

Prevention and Treatment Options

Lifestyle and Diet Tips

Mental exercises of all types help to keep the brain sharp (this is known as the use it or lose it theory). Reading, crossword puzzles, card games, and any other activity that requires the brain to exercise itself, so to speak, can help. Aerobic exercise also helps to keep the human blood vessels clean and to allow good blood flow to the brain. Check with your doctor to see if this is an option for you.

Dietary Supplements and Over-the-Counter Options

There is some research to suggest that fish oil or omega-3 fatty acids (EPA and DHA) and vitamin D can help reduce the risk of cognitive impairment. There is very little research on the herbal product ginkgo biloba, and it could overly thin your blood, so it is not recommended.

Prescriptions and Medical Procedures

There is some new preliminary research to suggest that low doses of estrogen may help prevent or treat this condition. Estrogen can also reduce bone loss in men on ADT, but it does carry an increased risk for causing blood clots.

CONSTIPATION

What is it? Why does it happen? Constipation is an acute or chronic condition in which bowel movements occur less often than usual or consist of hard, dry stools that are painful or difficult to pass. The intestines normally are active and moving in a wave-like motion (peristalsis), so that stools can move out of the body on a regular basis. If the wave-like motion slows, or too much water is removed from the intestines, the stools become drier, harder, and more difficult to pass.

Some drugs (Taxotere, for example) can increase intestinal movement or draw more water into the intestines and cause diarrhea, but other common products such as iron supplements or calcium carbonate dietary supplements slow intestinal movement and can cause constipation. Many medications (over 100 prescription medications and some over-the-counter products) can increase the risk of constipation, but it is especially common with stronger prescription pain medications, including:

- Codeine (with or without acetaminophen)
- Fentanyl
- Hydrocodone
- Hydromorphone
- Meperidine
- Methadone
- Morphine
- Oxycodone
- Oxymorphone
- Propoxyphene
- Tramadol

What are the signs/symptoms? Hard, difficult-to-pass bowel movements, straining to go, bloating, belly pain and cramping, and excess gas are all symptoms of constipation. Chronic constipation can increase the risk of several other conditions, including:

- Anal- and rectal-area cracks or breaks and potential infection
- Bleeding in the rectal area
- Fecal impaction (stool gets stuck in the intestines, a medical emergency)
- Hemorrhoids

Prevention and Treatment Options

Lifestyle and Diet Tips

- Exercise helps to stimulate digestion and keep things moving to prevent constipation. However, exercise can also be dehydrating, which can make constipation worse. If you are able to exercise regularly, please be sure to get plenty of fluids.
- In general, fluids (particularly water or low-calorie sports drinks) are your friend, because they will help to keep

stools soft.

- Foods that are high in fiber are important to help with regularity. Fiber helps to draw water into the intestines and stimulates the intestines to keep moving. (Your goal is to get 20–30 grams of fiber per day in your diet.) See below for some rich sources of fiber from many different food sources.
- Avoid regular or heavy use of very-low-fiber foods, such as highly processed food or meat, cheese, and eggs. These are sources of protein, but fiber can be added to your diet by selecting some alternative sources such as beans or nuts.
- Flaxseed and chia seeds (not the liquid or pills, but the seed or ground seeds) are good sources of fiber that can be added to many foods or beverages.
- Don't laugh, but chewing gum has been shown to help the bowels start or keep moving after surgery. It won't hurt to try some gum chewing to help keep the bowels moving during cancer treatment.

Dietary Supplements and Over-the-Counter Options

- Fiber pills are not terribly effective, and they can cost a lot of money because you have to take so many of them to reach your goal of 20 to 30 grams of fiber per day.
- Fiber powders and bars are okay, but they can't be outdone by fiber from foods. For example, 1/3 cup of All-Bran is inexpensive, and it contains a full 13 to 15 grams of fiber. It would take 4 or 5 cups of water, each with a rounded teaspoon of fiber powder, to equal that amount of fiber. Mix the bran

TOP SOURCES OF DIETARY FIBER	GRAMS OF FIBER
Vegetables	
Artichoke (1 whole, cooked)	10
Artichoke hearts (1 cup)	7
Parsnips (1 cup)	5.5
Broccoli (1 cup)	4.5
Brussels sprouts (1 cup)	4.5
Legumes and Beans	
Cranberry beans (2/3 cup)	12
Baked beans (1/2 cup)	9
Kidney beans (1/2 cup)	7-8
Split peas (1/2 cup)	6.7
Navy beans (1/2 cup)	6
Grains and Cereals	
Wheat-bran cereal (All-Bran, FiberOne) (1/3 cup)	10-14
Oatmeal (3/4 cup)	4-5
Bran Chex cereal (2/3 cup)	4.5
Raisin bran–type cereals	4
Spaghetti (whole wheat) (1/2 cup cooked)	4-6
Nuts and Seeds	
Flaxseed (golden) (2 tbsp.)	4–6
Chestnuts (10 roasted kernels)	4-5
Chia seeds (1 tbsp.)	4-5
Flaxseed (regular, brown) (2 tbsp.)	3-4
Almonds (5 nuts)	3-4
Sunflower seeds (1 oz.)	3-4

cereal with another cereal or with yogurt, and you've got a good fiber start to your day.
- Keep in mind that most healthy foods contain a mixture of insoluble and soluble fiber, but most contain insoluble fiber. For example, an apple is mostly insoluble fiber. However, most supplements, bars, and fiber powders are made of soluble fiber. Many people have trouble digesting a lot of soluble fiber, which means that fiber from food sources just makes more sense.
- When it comes to treating (not preventing) constipation, fiber supplements become more helpful, as do a variety of laxatives.

Over-the-Counter Constipation Treatments

The chart to the right lists a number of laxatives used for treating constipation if preventive measures are not adequate to provide relief. Keep in mind that laxatives should only be used for short amounts of time. It is important to allow the bowels to begin to pass stools more naturally on their own, as opposed to becoming dependent on laxatives.

Prescriptions and Medical Procedures

There are several prescription laxative treatments available. Ask your doctor about these if over-the-counter treatments are not working. For example, lubiprostone (Amitiza) is approved for chronic constipation; it softens the stool. Polyethylene glycol is an osmotic laxative that softens the stool by causing the stool to draw in and hold water. It is found over the counter and in a more potent prescription form. Lactulose (sold under many commercial names) is another prescription that brings in water to soften the stool.

DEPRESSION AND MOOD CHANGES

What is it? Why does it happen? Depression is a feeling of sadness or listless, a general lack of interest in life. Being diagnosed with cancer and going through any treatment can be a challenge to an individual both physically and mentally. Therefore, it is important to discuss mental health before,

Laxative Products and Their Action	**Examples** Always check for less expensive generic options.
Fiber Supplements and Bulk-Forming Laxatives work by absorbing or drawing water into the intestine to make the stool softer. These laxatives *must* be taken with water.	Citrucel Metamucil Fiber (generic)
Lubricant Laxatives work by lubricating the stool to allow it to move through the intestines more easily.	Mineral oil
Saline Laxatives and Osmotics work like a sponge to draw or attract water into the colon to make the stool softer.	Citrate of Magnesia Kristalose Magnesium citrate/salt (generics) Milk of Magnesia MiraLAX Phillips' M-O Polyethylene glycol (generic)
Stimulant Laxatives work by increasing the movement or activity of the intestines so that the muscles contract and keep stools moving forward.	Correctol Dulcolax Bisacodyl (generic) Ex-Lax Senokot Sennosides (generic) Castor oil
Stool Softeners work by moistening the stool to make it softer.	Colace Dialose Surfak Docusate (generic)

during, and especially after prostate cancer treatment of any kind. Whether you are waiting for the next PSA test, or trying to get into a clinical trial, or experiencing a new side effect, cancer can be stressful.

What are the signs or symptoms? The most common symptoms of depression in men include low self-esteem, suicidal thoughts, loss of interest in usually pleasurable activities, fatigue, changes in appetite, sleep disturbances, and apathy.

Prevention and Treatment Options

Lifestyle and Diet Tips

- Watch your diet. If your diet is well balanced, your body is more likely to feel good and function well.
- Check with your doctor to see what types of exercise you can do. Being active boosts your energy level and can also boost your mood.
- Get a proper amount of sleep—not too much, not too little. Lack of sleep can affect your mood greatly. Take short naps during the day if needed.
- Get outdoors in the sunlight each day, if possible. Sunlight affects chemical levels in the body and can help depression.
- Seek out stress-relieving activities such as writing in a journal, support groups, religious activities, or professional counseling. Discussing your situation with another person can improve your mental state.

Dietary Supplements and Over-the-Counter Options

There are some dietary supplements that look interesting, such as SAM-e (S-adenosylmethionine), omega-3 fatty acids, and fish oil pills. However, as we've cautioned before, patients undergoing cancer treatments need to be cautious and talk with their doctors before trying any new supplements.

One you should avoid: St. John's Wort is an herbal product that is often recommended for depression, and it may help. However, prostate cancer patients are strongly advised to stay away from this herbal product because it has been shown to reduce the effectiveness of many medications, including some cancer drugs.

Prescriptions and Medical Procedures
Many prescription medications are available and effective in helping patients cope with depression today. The most common medication classes are SSRIs and SNRIs, and some of these same medications have also been shown to reduce hot flashes. Talk to your doctor about the options.

DIARRHEA

What is it? Why does it happen? Diarrhea occurs when certain cancer treatments (radiation, certain drugs, or chemotherapy treatments) damage some of the healthy cells of the intestines. Another possible cause is suppression of immune cells during cancer treatment that allows an infection to develop in the gut, resulting in diarrhea. With diarrhea, the patient is not able to absorb enough water from the stool in the intestines because the lining of the intestine isn't working properly due to a cancer drug or infection.
What are the signs/symptoms? Loose or watery stools, several times a day, with or without discomfort or pain. Symptoms can include weight loss and even fever in some cases. Diarrhea is, in general, described by doctors in terms of its frequency and severity, in much the same way most other side effects are classified. Grade 1 and 2 are easier to control and treat, and Grade 3 and 4 represent more serious side effects. Diarrhea is more specifically defined in the following way as compared to your "normal" or "baseline."

- Grade 1: increase of up to 4 separate loose stool episodes per day above baseline
- Grade 2: increase of 4–6 loose stools per day, and/or need for IV fluids for less than 24 hours
- Grade 3: increase of 7 or more loose stools per day, not controllable/fecal incontinence, and need for IV fluids for more than 24 hours
- Grade 4: life-threatening

Basically, any diarrhea during the time of cancer treatment should be discussed with your doctor, just as with any other side effect. With any side effect, giving details to the doctor might seem uncomfortable, but it helps your doctor assess and treat your situation. For example, the number of times you are going to the bathroom per day, what the stools look like (dark, light, bloody), whether you have cramping or pain, nausea and vomiting, or even fever with the diarrhea are important details to report.

Diarrhea can lead to dehydration, electrolyte loss (key nutrient losses), inadequate nutrition, inflammation, bleeding, and pain. A severe case can also injure the intestines.

Prevention and Treatment Options

Lifestyle and Diet Tips

- You do not need to change your diet in anticipation of possible diarrhea. A patient on a potential drug that could cause diarrhea can eat a full, non-restricted diet. If diarrhea occurs, you should then avoid greasy, spicy, fatty, fried, and really sweet foods, because these foods can irritate the intestines while they are injured.
- You should avoid milk and milk products during and for a week or more after diarrhea occurs. The cancer drugs that cause diarrhea also can cause a temporary loss of the compound in the gut that helps to digest the sugar found in milk and dairy products (lactose), temporarily causing an intolerance to those products.
- Be careful about fiber during a bout of diarrhea, because high-fiber foods (beans, vegetables, fiber supplements) can draw more water into the intestines and actually make the diarrhea worse.
- Doctors often recommend a BRAT diet for diarrhea suffers. The BRAT letters stand for **B**ananas, **R**ice, **A**pplesauce, and **T**oast. Together with instructions to drink clear liquids, it is a good suggestion to treat diarrhea. A clear liquid is in general any type of liquid that you can see through or that is mostly made of water. For example, apple juice (no pulp) and water are clear liquids, but milk and orange juice (may have pulp) are not clear liquids. Here are some possible options if

you suffer from diarrhea:
  - Black coffee (no cream and sugar)
  - Ice chips
  - Fruit juice (no pulp, such as apple juice)
  - Jell-O (plain)
  - Pedialyte (electrolyte drinks that can be purchased at a grocery or drug store)
  - Popsicle (no fruit or pulp in it)
  - Soft drinks
  - Soup broth (liquid only, no solid ingredients)
  - Sports drinks (such as Gatorade or Powerade)
  - Tea (no cream and sugar)
  - Water
- Drinking fluids to hydrate your body is very important! Food intake during diarrhea is a less significant concern, but maintaining fluid intake is critical. Drinking lots of clear liquids helps make up for the large quantity of lost fluid with each diarrheal episode. Fluids should consist not just of plain water, but also electrolytes (important compounds to maintain health, such as magnesium and potassium), salt, and some minimal sugar daily to meet the needs of the human body.
- Be careful using sugar alcohol sweeteners that replace sugar, for example xylitol, mannitol, and sorbitol (note that they all end in "ol"). They can be usually found in candy and gum, and rarely also in some beverages and foods. When these sweeteners are swallowed they can cause cramping or abdominal pain, similar to some of the symptoms of diarrhea. The body usually develops tolerance to these sugar alcohol sweeteners over time, but they should be avoided particularly if you have diarrhea.
- When diarrhea begins to improve, your diet can be slowly expanded to add pasta (without sauce), white-meat chicken (without skin), scrambled eggs, and other easy-to-digest foods. Cruciferous vegetables, such as broccoli, Brussels sprouts, cauliflower, and cabbage should not be consumed initially because they

are very high in fiber and may produce gas, bloating, and intestinal cramping.

Dietary Supplements and Over-the-Counter Options

- Loperamide (Imodium A-D and generic options) is one of the most common and probably most effective over-the-counter drugs that can help reduce diarrhea, particularly grade 1 or 2. It is available as a pill or caplet, with each caplet having 2 mg of the medication. It works by slowing the movement of the gastrointestinal tract (reducing peristalsis), thus increasing the amount of time during which water can be absorbed in the gut. Patients generally take an initial 4 mg dosage, followed by 2 mg doses every 4 hours, or after each more uniform stool. The maximum dosage per day is 16 mg/day. This dose may be increased after consulting with your doctor in cases where the diarrhea is persisting beyond 24 hours. Loperamide can be continued for about 12 hours after your normal stools begin again and a normal diet has been restarted, just to ensure longer-term efficacy and that the problem with diarrhea has truly resolved. If you have trouble taking pills, Loperamide liquid (usually for kids) supplies about 1 mg of the medication for each 7.5 ml of the liquid and can also be used by adults.
- Other anti-diarrheal over-the-counter medications, such as bismuth subsalicylate (Pepto-Bismol, Kaopectate, or Maalox, for example) have not received as much research in the area of diarrhea from cancer treatment, so do not take these products without first talking to your doctor. Bismuth subsalicylate reduces the flow of fluids into the intestines, reduces inflammation and the overactive movement of the bowels, and can destroy organisms that can cause diarrhea or bind to the toxins that can cause diarrhea. This drug is turned into salicylic acid (similar to aspirin) in the gut, which is why it is effective at reducing inflammation and helping some patients. However, if you are allergic to aspirin or have been told not to take aspirin, you should stay away from these products. In addition, taking

bismuth subsalicylate products can turn your tongue and stools black temporarily in some patients. Be sure to check with your doctor if you are considering this option.

- Some preliminary laboratory studies of the amino acid glutamine shows that it may improve electrolyte absorption and nutrient movement during diarrhea that could be beneficial. However, the small number of clinical studies conducted so far have not been impressive enough to recommend using it as a regular treatment for diarrhea. However, using glutamine to prevent neuropathy (see the neuropathy section later in this chapter) may make more sense.
- In a small study of individuals receiving pelvic radiation for prostate cancer, low-dose psyllium fiber supplementation (Metamucil, for example) has been recommended at 1 to 2 teaspoons a day for the prevention and treatment of diarrhea. This represents only one study from a decade ago, and there has not been another publication to support or refute this finding. However, there is a low amount of fiber involved, so ask your doctor whether this should be considered in the case of radiation treatment. As mentioned earlier, fiber supplements should be avoided in most individuals suffering from diarrhea.
- Probiotics ("friendly" bacteria that can restore your normal gut bacteria) are getting a lot of attention to reduce diarrhea in children on antibiotics, but the research in preventing and treating diarrhea caused by cancer treatment is not adequate right now to make a recommendation. Since probiotics also have the chance of causing some harm in some patients, a safer recommendation may be to take some natural probiotics by eating plain white yogurt or a yogurt drink.
- Skin hygiene is important when you have diarrhea. Clean the skin area around the anus carefully and gently with warm water and a soft cloth regularly if you have diarrhea, because the skin around this area can

become irritated and painful. Another good option is to take a sitz bath and allow the warm water to relieve the discomfort and cleanse the area. You can obtain Epsom salts at a local pharmacy to add to the water. Epsom salts contain magnesium sulfate salts that are actually absorbed into the skin area during this bath.

Prescriptions and Medical Procedures

- Although it hasn't received a lot of attention in cancer treatment, diphenoxylate/atropine combinations (Lonox or Lomotil and others) seem to work similarly to loperamide by slowing down the movement of the gut to increase the amount of time during which water can be absorbed. This drug can be given or prescribed in combination with loperamide (the over-the-counter medication mentioned earlier). In general, patients take 1 or 2 tablets every 6 to 8 hours with loperamide. This drug combination does not work as well for severe diarrhea.
- Antibiotics are given in certain situations where there is persistent diarrhea that may be due to an infection. They may be prescribed for patients having a low white blood cell count (neutropenia).
- Rifaximin (Xifaxan) is a non-systemic antibiotic, which means that very little of the drug will ever leave the gastrointestinal tract. This has become a popular drug for preventing and treating traveler's diarrhea caused by E. coli bacteria, and now it seems to be showing some efficacy for other bowel conditions such as irritable bowel syndrome (IBS), and even inflammation of the portions of the bowel (diverticulitis). This drug has few side effects and has a low risk of causing resistance. It is unknown at this time whether it might play a role in treating diarrhea from chemotherapy.
- Octreotide (Sandostatin) is a hormone-like drug that gets some attention on the Internet and has been used for reducing diarrhea from gastrointestinal cancers. It has not been tested in HRPC, but it is a possible option to discuss with your doctor if there is a lack of other options

available for severe diarrhea that is not improving with other therapies. This drug may slow the movement of the intestines and allow more water to be absorbed out of the intestines. The drug comes in several versions and can be given as an injection, IV drug, or as a pill.

- If someone is hospitalized because of diarrhea (rarely with grade 4), doctors have multiple options (IV fluids, strong medications, etc.) available to control and resolve the problem. Since hospitalization is rare, we won't spend more time on those options in this book.

DRY SKIN AND DERMATITIS

What is it? Why does it happen? Dermatitis refers to irritation of the skin. Some men complain of dry skin issues when they are given long-term ADT or certain other testosterone-changing medications. This seems to make sense if you think about menopause and women for a moment. When women lose estrogen over several years (and experience menopause), they are more likely to experience dry skin. Men undergoing ADT experience a male menopause in about one to three months. So, dry skin can also be an issue that needs to be discussed.

What are the signs or symptoms? Dry, flaking, or irritated skin.

Prevention and Treatment Options

Lifestyle and Diet Tips

There are plenty of inexpensive and simple options for preventing and treating dry skin.

- Dry air, cold air, indoor heating, friction, and even heavy clothing can make your skin dry, itchy, red, and easily cracked.
- Long hot showers and baths are not a good idea. Hot water removes the natural oils that the skin produces. ADT or not, as you get older your body produces less and less protective skin oil.
- Do not use antibacterial, deodorant, or perfumed soaps, which can cause drying. Use a mild, moisturizing, and scent-free cleanser.

- Use warm rather than hot water.
- Keep the bathroom door closed to keep in the humidity, and do not dry your skin aggressively with a towel after the shower or bath because your skin needs to be a little wet when applying moisturizer.
- Use moisturizer early and often when the air is dry in the fall and winter months. A moisturizer right after a shower in the morning is perhaps the best way to protect your skin. Use a product with glycerin, petrolatum (Vaseline), fatty acids (stearic acid, for example), ceramide, or cholesterol while your skin is still slightly damp. Reapply during the day as needed.
- During warm and humid months, use moisturizer more sparingly to allow moisture from the air to reach your skin.
- If you use a facial moisturizer, as most people should (including men), please use a broad-spectrum (UVA- and UVB-blocker) product with an SPF of at least 15 to 30.
- Increase the humidity in your house. You can put a water-filled bowl near a radiator or heating vent, fill the bathtub, or just use a humidifier. Look for a device that has a humidistat, which is a control that automatically shuts off the device when the target humidity is reached.
- Do not use electric blankets unless it is really needed, because they remove moisture from the skin.
- Wear soft clothes and try to avoid wool and other rough fabrics. Try to wear cotton or silk next to your skin, and use an unscented fabric softener to avoid chemicals and perfumes that can cause excess drying.
- Use lip moisturizer with an SPF of 15 or more in it, or even petroleum jelly if you need it.
- You can treat cracked heels with moisturizers with lactic acid or urea, and cotton-lined plastic or rubber gloves are a good way to go when washing dishes.

Dietary Supplements and Over-the-Counter Options

None needed.

Prescriptions and Medical Procedures

None needed.

ERECTILE DYSFUNCTION AND LOSS OF LIBIDO

Also known as ED

What is it? Why does it happen? Erectile dysfunction (ED) is an inability to get or maintain an erection adequate enough for sexual activity or sexual intercourse. A loss of libido simply means feeling uninterested in sexual activity. Most prostate cancer treatments may cause some degree of ED and/or libido problems. It makes sense that treatments that affect the levels of the male hormone testosterone would also impact sexuality. In general, localized prostate cancer treatment (surgery, radiation, cryotherapy) has traditionally been associated with some ED, and ADT or hormone manipulation has been associated with a loss of libido.

What are the signs or symptoms? ED can take days, weeks, or months after prostate cancer treatment to occur. Some doctors are encouraging patients to use a variety of ED treatment options (pills, pumps, etc.) soon after treatment to help reduce the risk of future ED problems. Talk to your doctor about this more aggressive treatment option, now known as penile rehabilitation.

Prevention and Treatment Options

Lifestyle and Diet Tips

Generally speaking, things that are heart healthy are also positive steps to take for sexual health and maintaining an erection. Exercise, controlling blood pressure, cholesterol lowering, weight loss … all can help to improve blood flow to the penis.

Dietary Supplements and Over-the-Counter Options

The chart on the following page will give you some ideas of supplements that may possibly help. As we have cautioned repeatedly for cancer patients, always check with your doctor before taking any new medication or supplement, for it may interfere with your ongoing treatment or be unsafe for your condition.

Type of Therapy	**Korean red ginseng** (1,500–3,000 mg/day) has helped some men with ED **MACA** (1500–3000 mg/day)
Advantages	Cost-effective dietary supplements Numerous small published clinical trials. May improve libido/sex drive (including LHRH patients).
Disadvantages	Minimal research in prostate cancer patients Minimal research on long-term safety (use it at your own risk). Other supplements may be very dangerous. L-arginine in high doses may cause cardiovascular problems in some patients from a recent large clinical trial. Quality control issues.

Prescriptions and Medical Procedures

The following are options to discuss with your doctor.

Type of Therapy	**Orally ingested phosphodiesterase inhibitors** (also known as "PDE-5 inhibitors")
Advantages	Pills taken by mouth. Effective for most men.
Disadvantages	Not effective in patients who have had prostatectomy, unless some nerve-sparing approach was used. Side effects include headache, nasal congestion, and muscle and back pain. Can be expensive. 30–60 minutes wait for response.

Disadvantages (continued)	Cannot be taken with some medications. No impact on low libido (sex drive).
Type of Therapy	**Intra-urethral suppository** (common doses available 125, 250, 500, and 1000 mcg).
Advantages	Small pellet placed in the urethra without needles. Few systemic side effects. Effective in some men.
Disadvantages	Can cause penile pain. Requires training. Can be expensive. Side effects include (rarely) painful and prolonged erection of more than 4 hours, fainting, dizziness.
Type of Therapy	**Penile injection** (multiple doses and options available, such as Bimix and Trimix, check with your doctor).
Advantages	Highly effective. Few systemic side effects. Works in three to five minutes.
Disadvantages	Requires injection. Requires office training. Can be expensive. Can cause penile pain. Can cause prolonged erection and penile scars or fibrosis.

Type of Therapy	Vacuum device
Advantages	Least expensive. No systemic side effects. Effective in most patients. Battery-operated option now available.
Disadvantages	Can cause numbness or bruising. Less "natural" erection. Trapped ejaculate. May be awkward to use.
Type of Therapy	**Penile prosthesis**
Advantages	Highly effective. For men who have failed or are not satisfied with medical treatment of ED.
Disadvantages	Small risk of infection. Requires anesthesia and surgery. May require replacement after many years of u

FATIGUE

Also known as asthenia, weakness, or lack of energy and strength.

What is it? Why does it happen? This is a common side effect of most advanced cancer treatments. The risk of fatigue increases the longer a patient is being treated with a certain cancer drug, such as chemotherapy. Cancer treatments can reduce blood counts that are important in maintaining energy levels, and being exposed to higher doses of certain drugs simply depletes or reduces numerous compounds in the body that can help maintain energy levels. Other causes of fatigue include hormonal reductions or changes from treatment (thyroid hormones and testosterone, for example), pain and its possible impact on sleep, a lack of adequate nutrition, and other side effects such as nausea and vomiting. Also, mental fatigue (depression, stress, and anxiety) can lead to physical fatigue, and vice versa. Both mental and physical fatigue are not uncommon during a long cancer treatment process. For all these reasons, it is important for you and your doctor to determine the true cause of your fatigue because it may or may not actually be drug related.

What are the signs or symptoms? Patients offer many different descriptions, but they all revolve around a lack of energy. Examples are fatigue, weakness, reduced energy and strength, daily lack of energy, and whole-body tiredness that is not improved by sleep or excessive resting periods. If you are spending a good share of your days in bed or in a chair, it is time to talk to your doctor about potentially having your fatigue treated.

Prevention and Treatment Options

Lifestyle and Diet Tips

- Exercise (aerobic and weightlifting) has been shown in numerous clinical trials to improve energy levels and reduce fatigue. In fact, weight lifting in prostate cancer patients has continued to show excellent results. However, keep in mind that a weightlifting regimen should not be attempted without the approval of your doctor because men with bone metastasis can injure themselves or suffer a fracture while weightlifting.
- Aerobic exercise every other day (biking, jogging, rowing, soccer, and swimming) is generally recommended because it takes the body longer to recover from exercise during cancer treatment. This means that if you are experiencing more severe fatigue and exercising almost daily it is perhaps time to cut back on your exercise regimen to allow your body a longer recovery period. Most clinical studies of exercise ask patients to work out only 2 or 3 days a week. Optimally, try to include aerobic exercise every other day for approximately 30 minutes, and on the other days (rest days) feel free to perform light activity such as a short walk. This should help keep you at your peak mental and physical health. As always, consult with your doctor to see if this fits for your particular health situation.

- Talk to a nutritionist about calculating an adequate daily calorie count and establishing a nutritional balance during cancer treatment. Your caloric needs are approximately 15 calories per pound that you carry, on average. This means that a person who weighs 150 pounds needs about 2250 calories per day to maintain weight. Using the same calculation, a person who weighs 200 pounds needs 3000 calories to maintain weight. And every single pound of unwanted weight loss during cancer treatment means that you need to add about 500 calories per day to try to get it back over several weeks.
- High-quality proteins are needed for rebuilding and repairing body tissues and are also a good source of energy. The best high-quality protein comes from dairy, eggs, fish, meat, and poultry. If you do not eat some of these things, there are also whey protein and egg protein powders (just add water), and soy protein. For complete vegetarians or vegans, there are newer soy protein and brown rice protein powders that are high-quality protein sources, just not as good as the animal sources of protein. Protein requirements on average are about 0.8 grams of total protein per kilogram of body weight (1 kilogram=2.2 pounds). This means a 150-pound (68-kilogram) person needs about 54 grams of protein a day. However, a 200-pound (91-kilogram) person needs about 73 grams of protein a day. This might initially sound like a lot, but a small protein drink and a small serving (mini-can) of tuna fish give you about 40 to 50 grams of protein. Nuts, seeds, and soy all have more than 10 grams in a small serving. Some common sources of protein are listed here.

GRAMS OF PROTEIN	
Steak	40
Chicken breast	30
Fish (3 oz.)	20
Protein Powder (1 serving)	15 to 20
Eggs (2)	12 to 15
Milk (1 cup)	8
Yogurt (1 cup)	8

- Caffeine is a wonderful and healthy-in-moderation compound to help reduce fatigue. In general, green or black tea has about one third to one half the amount of caffeine of a cup of coffee. Coffee, tea, a soda or diet soda with caffeine—all are perfectly fine. Several servings a day are considered usually safe and effective. Be careful not to consume these products late in the day or in the early evening because they can promote restlessness and a lack of adequate sleep. Caffeine has also recently been shown to help muscles recover from exercise, which can also help improve your overall energy levels.

- In general, caffeine pills, energy drinks, or energy shots are not recommended for cancer fatigue. Because these caffeine doses are very concentrated and high, they can cause jitters, nervousness, and added stress. Also, patients can build a tolerance whereby much larger doses are needed over time to have any effect. Finally, withdrawal from these very high doses of caffeine provided by pills and energy drinks is tough and often can cause moderate to severe headaches.
- Yerba mate and guarana should be considered synonyms for the word "caffeine". These are found in some beverages, and they are actually plants or derivatives from plants that have caffeine in them. Be careful to consider them as you would other caffeine products. They can give you all the advantages (reduce fatigue) and disadvantages (sleeplessness, jitters, heart rate increases) of increased caffeine intake, because they offer basically the same thing.

Dietary Supplements and Over-the-Counter Options

- American Ginseng (Panax quinquefolius) and perhaps Korean Ginseng (Panax ginseng) are now backed by clinical research (particularly American ginseng) from a large randomized trial that suggests that 1000 to 2000 mg a day dosages given as a pill can reduce cancer treatment–related fatigue. This is very exciting and should be discussed with your doctor. The study was very well done. Ginseng is arguably the best potential dietary supplement for fatigue for cancer patients as compared to any other dietary supplement, simply based on the large amount of research.
- Ribose is a natural sugar produced by the body that can

also be purchased at health food stores as a powder to put into beverages. Ribose (or D-Ribose) can also be purchased as a pill. There have been a few preliminary studies (not nearly as comprehensive as the ginseng studies) that suggest that patients taking 5 grams with a beverage at breakfast, lunch, and dinner (15 grams a day total) experience a reduction in chronic fatigue from unknown causes. The supplement has a good safety record and may be worth trying for a week or two. As always, check with your doctor before taking any supplements to see if they are a good idea for your individual situation.

- L-carnitine is a dietary supplement that has excited lots of researchers because it makes sense that it might work to reduce cancer-related fatigue. L-carnitine is a compound that exists in the human body to transport other compounds into every cell so that more energy can be produced. However, the clinical trials have not borne out all the hype, so researchers are not sure how well these supplements really work for cancer fatigue. There have been a few small studies to suggest that getting 1 to 2 grams (1000 to 2000 mg) per day of L-carnitine supplements or pills may reduce cancer fatigue in some individuals. Check with your doctor, because trying this option makes sense only if other things don't work.

Prescriptions and Medical Procedures

- Armodafinil (Nuvigil) is an oral drug used by some doctors to reduce fatigue from cancer treatment. It tends to work by stimulating areas of the brain that promote wakefulness or being awake, and it can be given once daily (150 or 250 mg per day in the morning). It is also used to keep awake individuals who have an abnormal condition that makes them fall asleep easily even after getting enough sleep. It has been used illegally by students to pull "all-nighters" before a test. The drug can cause headache, nausea, and dizziness, but perhaps the biggest side effect is not being able to get to sleep (insomnia). For this reason, the drug is taken in the morning as opposed to later in the day. This drug is similar in its action to the drug modafanil (Provigil), but armodafanil seems to stay in the body longer and may be more effective in reducing fatigue.

- Other prescription stimulant medications (methylphenidate, for one) that are prescribed for other purposes (ADHD, for example) are undergoing some good research to help treat fatigue.
- GM-CSF, used to prevent infections and also known as Leukine and other names, helps to reduce weakness because it helps to maintain an adequate blood count. Low blood counts can drain energy from the body.
- Anti-depressive medications have been tested in several trials to determine whether they can reduce cancer-related fatigue, and they have not been successful.
- Because, as we discussed earlier, there are so many causes of low energy levels, it is best to work directly with your doctor to determine the cause in your case and then find the most appropriate medication.

FEVER

It is recommended that all men being treated for HRPC purchase an easy-to-read digital thermometer. It can be used to determine if they are experiencing fever following a treatment. With some treatments, such as Provenge, slight fever could be a temporary reaction to the immune therapy, but in other cases fever could be an indicator of a low immune cell count (neutropenia) that can occur after chemotherapy treatment. It is important to understand what is expected with your treatment and to talk with your physician if you have a fever. Your doctor may recommend acetaminophen use if she or he determines that the fever is only a mild and temporary reaction.

FLUID RETENTION

Also known as peripheral edema or lymphedema.

What is it? Why does it happen? It is always possible, although rare, that a person may experience mild or moderate fluid retention when receiving a new cancer treatment. Usually this results from a drug or, at times, even from treatment such as radiation. Fluid generally builds up in the lower legs or lower arms (the peripheral areas of the body). This can also happen in rare situations after patients have been on certain treatments, such as chemotherapy, for a long time. The longer a treatment time with a drug, the higher the risk of fluid retention.

Fluid retention occurs when the network of vessels that carries fluid away from the extremities is not functioning normally due to some form of toxicity. When lymph nodes (drainage areas for this fluid) are removed or injured during treatment, an individual loses some of his drainage capacity, and fluid can accumulate in the areas where the lymph nodes were injured or removed. If you think about it, the human body is amazingly good at making sure that fluid does not normally accumulate in the feet or ankles: fluid and even blood have to work their way up the body, against gravity, to get back to the heart so that they can be properly circulated and filtered. It is understandable, then, how any small damage to the vessels that carry fluid can cause fluid retention.

What are the signs or symptoms? Swelling in the ankles and feet, and less often the arms and hands, is one of the most common indications that there is fluid retention. In general, the feet and ankles do not appear to be a different color but just larger in shape. In the early stages it might not even be very noticeable, but with more time, it may be apparent just when putting on socks or shoes. Fluid retention can also occur in other parts of the body, such as the belly area. Weight gain can even be a sign of fluid retention. In more advanced stages, the patient may find it more difficult to breathe. The good news, as with many side effects in this book, is that steroid medications are usually given along with most cancer treatments today to reduce the risk of fluid retention.

- Oddly enough, motion is a leading preventive technique for edema. Keeping your body moving aids in circulation and improves edema. If possible, avoid sitting or standing for a long period of time, including when in the car or flying. Be sure to stretch your legs regularly.
- There is a concern that exercise and weightlifting can make fluid retention worse, but this has never really been proven. In breast cancer, at least, this hypothesis has been tested and disproven. Considering that exercise helps to keep you mentally and physically healthy during cancer treatment, it seems to make sense to keep moving. Maintaining aerobic exercise is important, and lifting weights is important. As we've discussed previously, remember to first get the okay from your doctor, because weightlifting or rigorous exercise may be a problem if there are bone metatases that can hurt or fracture the bone itself.
- Weigh yourself about once a week during cancer treatment. Chemotherapy, such as Taxotere, can be associated with some weight loss. Therefore, it is important to report to your doctor even a small gain in weight (2 to 4 pounds) because it may be caused by fluid retention.
- Pay attention to your fingers, ankles, and belly area for any sign of fluid accumulation. Report any difficulty in breathing or shortness of breath to your doctor.
- If you develop some peripheral edema, elevate the area, if you can. Let gravity help remove excess fluids from legs particularly. Your doctor may suggest you purchase support stockings at the pharmacy or drug store.
- Follow a low-salt diet (less than 2400 mg per day at a minimum, or ideally less than 1500 mg per day). Remember that the salt you ingest comes mostly from processed foods—canned, bagged, or boxed—not the salt shaker. If there is excess salt in the body, you may have trouble improving your edema.

Dietary Supplements and Over-the-Counter Options

Various dietary supplements are touted to prevent and possibly treat fluid retention. One such herbal supplement is "horse chestnut" (Aesculus hippocastanum), which has the active ingredient aescin (or escin). However, apart from breast cancer, where lymphedema can occur, and for the treatment of varicose veins and hemorrhoids, this supplement has really not received much attention in relation to HRPC. You can talk to your doctor to see whether he or she feels it has a role in edema treatment or prevention, but it is generally accepted that the steroid prescription medications work better to prevent fluid retention than any over-the-counter product.

Prescriptions and Medical Procedures

- Steroid (corticosteroid) treatments such as prednisone and dexamethasone are given along with chemotherapy because they can reduce the risk of numerous side effects, including fluid retention. They work so well that fluid retention does not become a serious side effect for most patients.
- If fluid retention does occur, your doctor can give you a variety of medications to resolve it, including a class of medications known as diuretics. These diuretics help to move fluid out of the body into the urine. Treatment of fluid retention is time sensitive; the earlier the treatment, the more effective the result. For that reason, talk with your doctor if you have concerns about fluid retention.

HAIR LOSS

Also known as chemotherapy-induced alopecia (CIA) or anagen effluvium.

What is it? Why does it happen? There are three major and most frequent side effects of chemotherapy drugs, namely bone marrow suppression impacts (with fewer blood cells produced), gastrointestinal problems, and hair loss. All three occur because chemotherapy is toxic to the most rapidly dividing cells of the human body (cancer cells among them).

Unfortunately, other healthy rapidly dividing cells of the bone marrow, gastrointestinal tract, and hair follicles suffer some temporary and, at times, permanent damage as well.

What are the signs and symptoms? Hair shedding can occur as early as 1 to 3 weeks, or even several months after chemotherapy has been initiated. The hair loss tends to occur in multiple areas over the whole scalp and is known as diffuse hair loss. It isn't possible to predict how much hair will be lost.

CIA is usually temporary, with hair regrowth usually occurring 3 to 6 months after chemotherapy is stopped. The scalp is the most common area of hair loss. However, if chemotherapy is given in high doses for a long time, hair loss can occur in other areas including under the arms, eyebrows, eyelashes, pubic hair, and beard. In some individuals the regrown hair shows a change in color and/or feel or texture. The thickness of the hair may be reduced.

Following is a list of drugs by their tendency to cause hair loss. Please note that the major chemotherapy drug approved for HRPC patients (Taxotere) and other drugs commonly used in prostate cancer treatment often cause some hair loss.

DRUGS THAT COMMONLY CAUSE HAIR LOSS	DRUGS THAT SOMETIMES CAUSE HAIR LOSS	DRUGS THAT RARELY CAUSE HAIR LOSS
Adriamycin	Amsacrine	Capecitabine
Cyclophosphamide	Bleomycin	Carboplatin
Daunorubicin	Busulfan	Carmustine
Docetaxel (Taxotere)	Cabazitaxel (Jevtana)	Cisplatin
Ifosfamide	Cytarabine	Fludarabine
Epirubicin	5-fluorouracil	Methotrexate
Etoposide	Gemcitabine	Mitomycin C
Irinotecan	Lomustine	Mitroxantrone
Paclitaxel	Thiotepa	Procarbazine
Topotecan	Vinblastine	6-mercaptopurine
Vindesine	Vincristine	Raltritrexate
Vinorelbine		Streptozotocin

Prevention and Treatment Options

Lifestyle and Diet Tips

- Any pill, liquid, or procedure that has helped with genetic male or female pattern hair loss may have some potential application for CIA. Check with your doctor.

- Hairpieces are used by some patients and come in a variety of options for those interested.
- Baseball caps or other hats are another option, and so is simply shaving your head. Patients often say how empowering accepting the hair loss is, but the decision should be up to you. Do be sure to remember to use a hat or sunblock for hairless heads to avoid painful sunburns.

Dietary Supplements and Over-the-Counter Options

- A 2% minoxidil topical solution (generic now, formerly exclusively known as Rogaine) has shown some success in reducing the impact of hair loss when applied twice a day.
- There is now a 5% minoxidil solution available that may be a better option. The drug is usually applied with a plastic applicator and rubbed on the scalp with your fingers several times a day when the scalp is dry. It is important to thoroughly wash your hands with soap and/or an alcohol-based hand gel when you are finished applying the minoxidil because the medication could be further absorbed into your body, or by others who come into contact with your hands. Also, these medications are alcohol-based and can irritate or dry out the scalp.
- Some patients use certain shampoos to make the hair appear more dense and fuller. Although they have not been tested on CIA, they have been used for genetic male pattern hair loss for years. Some options include ketoconazole (2%) or pyrithione zinc (1%) shampoos, which are basically strong anti-dandruff shampoos. These shampoos do have the potential to increase hair density and size and increase the number of hair follicles that go into the growth (anagen) stage. They are generally used several times a week and rotated with your regular shampoo. Other shampoos that have been promoted to provide a fuller appearance can be utilized as well. They always rely on an effective cleaning agent (for example lauryl or laureth sulfate) and a thickening agent (stearic acid or another fat).

Some home remedies use a thickening oil on the hair, such as a small amount of coconut oil, but there is no research to support their use, and they can be quite messy.

- There are over-the-counter sprays and powders (Toppik, for one) that contain natural keratin protein fibers (similar to protein in hair). They do thicken thinning hair when used on certain areas of the scalp. Some of these options can work well, but determine which ones should be based on trial and error. Some of the cheaper products or imitations on the market can be quite messy when you are washing them out or sweating.
- There are also some small studies of saw palmetto or components of saw palmetto (saturated fatty acids, lauric acid, myristic acid) showing that they may slightly help hair growth. This herbal supplement is working in a somewhat similar way to the drug finasteride, but nowhere near as strong as that class of drug. However, these small studies involved men with hair loss from male pattern baldness (genetic) and not from chemotherapy. Many of the hair-growing "tonics" sold over the counter in pills to men and women actually contain saw palmetto or ingredients found in some of these herbs that may somewhat mimic the impact of prescription drugs such as finasteride (see page 157).
- There is some minimal research on vitamin D supplements and prescription medications to prevent hair loss from chemotherapy and to promote hair growth during and after chemotherapy. These studies show that vitamin D is needed either to put hair follicles in the growth stage or to prevent the hair from toxicity. Vitamin D is an important consideration for cancer patients, especially those on LHRH treatment for preventing bone loss, so hair growth might just be a side bonus. The downside of vitamin D supplements is the potential to overdose on them and to raise your blood

level of the vitamin too high. It is not recommended that clinicians take vitamin D blood levels far beyond 40 ng/ml (100 nmol/L), because the effects have not been studied. There is some evidence to suggest that more vitamin D is not better for prostate cancer patients.

- The only other dietary supplement being studied in the laboratory for CIA is N-acetylcysteine, but it is too early to tell whether this supplement does anything positive in this area.
- Laser light therapy combs are selling well in various countries around the world. Treatment requires that several times a week, for 10 to 15 minutes, you run the bulky comb-like device through your hair. There is some minimal research to suggest that it may increase blood flow to the scalp and promote hair growth. However, there are no good published studies on chemotherapy patients, and the devices can be very expensive, so be careful here.
- B vitamins (B1, B2, B6, B12, folic acid, pantothenic acid) and other dietary supplements are often advertised to help promote healthy hair by numerous supplement companies. It is important to emphasize that you should not use these compounds in excessive dosages beyond what could be found in a multivitamin. It is believed that excess amounts of these vitamins may stimulate tumor growth in patients with advanced cancer as much as they stimulate hair growth. These vitamins or minerals work not just by providing nutrients to the hair but also by bringing them to all cells of the human body. They work very differently from the more effective prescription drugs or skin treatments.
- On another hair-related topic, some patients have questioned the safety of the chemicals in hair dye. There seems to be little or no concern over using hair dye during and after your cancer treatment. In addition, dye arguably can improve the quality of life for someone

dealing with physical changes during or after treatment. There will never be enough research on this subject to make someone feel completely comfortable about using hair dye, but the slight concern over these products focuses mostly on the more permanent dyes and pertains to individuals who are exposed to these products on a consistent basis (those who work in the hair care industry).

- Lastly, some hair loss supplements simply contain a series of exotic herbs. They may be a concern because we have no idea about the safety or the potential interaction of these supplements with conventional treatment. Go carefully here!

Prescriptions and Medical Procedures

- No drugs are currently approved for the prevention or treatment of CIA.
- The only prescription pill approved for male hair loss is finasteride (Propecia), taken 1 mg daily, but this has not been tested in men with CIA. This does not mean that it will not help, but just that it needs more testing. Some men are already taking this drug at a larger 5 mg daily dose (formerly known exclusively as Proscar), or taking a similar drug dutasteride (Avodart), at a 0.5 mg daily dose for non-cancerous prostate enlargement (BPH), and it also helps promote hair growth in these situations. Some doctors do not mind if their patients are taking these drugs before, during, or after chemotherapy, while others think they could interfere with treatment or may lower the PSA artificially (this is controversial). Please ask your doctor about any of these pills if you are interested.
- Scalp-cooling procedures have been used experimentally in some medical centers since the 1970s. Scalp cooling is accomplished either with cooling agents applied with a cooling cap that is changed several times during each session, or just by regular cooling of the scalp with cold air or liquid. Some health care professionals think that

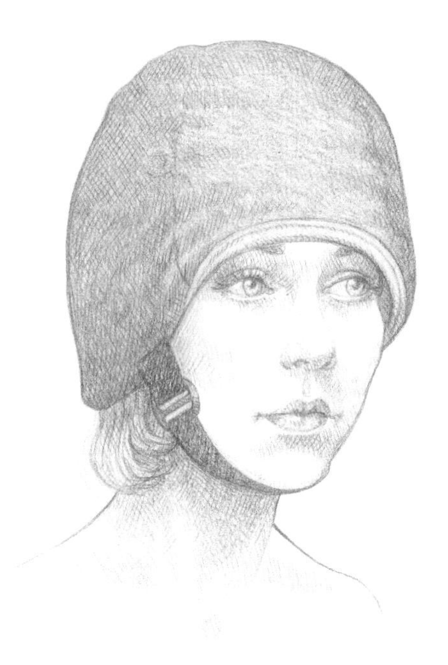

A cooling cap is used in some medical centers for male and female patients concerned with hair loss while undergoing chemotherapy.

scalp cooling may help because it makes the blood vessels in the scalp constrict. This reduces blood flow to the hair follicle during the time the patient is exposed to the highest amounts of the chemotherapy drug, thus reducing the amount of chemotherapy drug that can injure the hair itself. Others believe that scalp cooling puts the hair cells into a suspended state or reduces metabolic activity and makes them less vulnerable to a toxic agent. However, the catch on scalp cooling is that most published studies have not given detailed or very specific descriptions on the method used. For example, what is the appropriate length of time needed for best results? Potential side effects of scalp cooling include headaches, coldness and discomfort complaints, and anxiety from being around or in a small space (claustrophobia). If you are interested in scalp cooling, talk to your doctor—this should be done under clinical supervision and at specific times.

- Hair transplants are not advised for hair loss because this procedure works by taking hair that is genetically

programmed to not fall out from the back or sides of the head and transferring it to the areas of more permanent hair loss. This does not make sense when the hair loss is from chemotherapy because these hairs will also fall out.
- There is also a new drug approved to make eyelashes grow longer (Latisse or bimatoprost ophthalmic solution—0.03%). Some patients have asked whether they can use it if their eyelashes have been affected by chemotherapy (alopecia of the eyelashes). This drug has not been tested in patients receiving chemotherapy, and this particular side effect is rare. However, there are some published case reports of the medication helping some patients who have eyelash loss from other causes.

HOT FLASHES

Also known as hot flushes.

What is it? Why does it happen? Sudden, at times dramatic, feeling of heat, which may last seconds or minutes. Hot flashes may occur regularly throughout the day or only once in a while. Any treatment that reduces male hormone levels (ADT) can cause hot flashes, but the frequency and severity of hot flashes vary dramatically from one individual to another.

What are the signs and symptoms? By following the steps in this section, you will become more familiar with how serious your hot flashes are and whether or not they should be treated by conventional or alternative treatment, or just be tolerated. In hot flash clinical trials, most patients responded to some type of minimal intervention, but some patients can experience hot flashes that do not respond to simple lifestyle changes. For most mild to moderate hot flashes, a prescription drug is not needed, but for moderate to severe hot flashes, a prescription drug is usually needed. In the past, most men received prescription medical treatment for hot flashes, but recent clinical research suggests that only 20 to 30 percent of men need or ask for such medication. However, if you do need some help, prescription hot flash-reducing medications (especially progesterone pills and injections) work very well. Researchers have learned from studies of women going through menopause that lifestyle changes may play a large role in the management of hot flashes. Before deciding with your doctor about the proper treatment for your hot flashes, you need to determine the frequency and severity of the hot flashes.

Using the rating scale below, you can assess the situation with your hot flashes. Just photocopy the journal page that follows and use it to record your hot flash history for discussion with your doctor at your next visit. You may notice certain foods or activities that intensify the hot flashes and be able to make lifestyle changes that alleviate some of the occurrences.

SEVERITY	SCORE	LENGTH/ DURATION	OBSERVATIONS
MILD Hot Flash	1 point	Less than 1 minute	Warm & slightly uncomfortable, no perspiration
MODERATE Hot Flash	2 points	Less than 5 minutes	Warmth involving more of the body, perspiration, taking off some layers of clothing
SEVERE Hot Flash	3 points	Greater than 5 minutes	Burning warmth, disruption of normal life activities such as sleep or work, excessive perspiration, frequent thermostat changes in your house
VERY SEVERE Hot Flash	4 points	Time is not an issue	Complete disruption of normal activities to the point where it would make you consider discontinuing cancer drug treatment

PERSONAL HOT FLASH DIARY

Date: ______________________

Day of the Week: ______________________

Mild = 1 point
Moderate = 2 points
Severe = 3 points
Very Severe = 4 points

Time of Day	Severity of Hot Flash (Mild, Moderate, Severe or Very Severe)	Points	Activity During Hot Flash

Number of daily hot flashes: ______________________

Average severity: ______________________

Note on occurrences: ______________________

Prevention and Treatment Options

Lifestyle and Diet Tips

These remedies are the treatment of first choice, along with alternative medicines, for most men. By using the hot flash diary and some of the following low-cost lifestyle options, you may expect to see a 25 to 50 percent reduction overall in those annoying hot flashes. These methods are not sufficient for severe hot flashes, so we'll discuss prescription alternatives later.

Lifestyle Change	Advantages & Disadvantages
Avoid hot beverages, spicy foods, and excess alcohol or caffeine	Many foods and beverages can trigger hot flashes or make them worse. Your diary may help identify offenders for you.
Controlled, deep, slow abdominal breathing (6–8 breaths per minute) for at least 15 minutes twice daily (morning, midday and/or evening) or at the beginning of a hot flash	Also known as "paced respiration," it has been shown to decrease blood pressure (temporarily), hot flashes, and the severity of a hot flash. However, this technique needs practice or it may need to be taught to you because it involves moving stomach muscles in and out.
Keeping a diary	Diary-keeping for just 1 to 2 weeks can give you the best insight into what does and does not impact your hot flashes. Give it a try!
Avoid smoking or breathing secondhand smoke	Not only heart unhealthy, tobacco smoke makes hot flashes worse due to circulatory and temperature changes it produces in your body.
Low-impact daily exercise	Exercise has been shown to reduce stress and improve mood, and it may reduce hot flashes. Use a fan or work out in a cool location.
Stress reduction (meditation, relaxation techniques, yoga, etc.)	Relaxation exercises can help with flashes and may also improve other areas of your life, such as sleep.

Lifestyle Change	Advantages & Disadvantages
Use cooling methods—ice cubes, cool beverages, a fan that reduces room temperature, opening a window, chilling pillows and/or pillow coverings	If your body's core temperature increases slightly it can trigger a hot flash, so it just makes sense to keep yourself a bit cooler.
Wear loose-fitting clothing and layer clothing	Helps to keep your body's core temperature slightly lower, and prevents clothing from feeling constricting when a hot flash occurs. Layers allow you to easily shed clothing to regulate temperature shifts.

Dietary Supplements and Over-the-Counter Options

Along with the lifestyle changes discussed, these treatments are the best options for most men. It may be best to begin these prior to testosterone suppression, but you should check with your doctor before starting any treatment to be sure that they do not interfere with your cancer therapy. You should not consider more than one or two of these options at one time. As with the lifestyle changes, you may expect to see a 25 to 50 percent improvement using these treatments.

Complementary & Alternative Treatments	Advantages & Disadvantages
Acupuncture (1 to 2 times every week or two)	Few or no side effects; traditional needle and other forms of acupuncture have helped; can be costly.
Black cohosh pills (1 to 2 pills a day)	Moderate to expensive in price. Most research has been with women and shown it to work similar to a placebo.
Fish oil pills (at least 1200 mg a day total of EPA & DHA—the active ingredients)	Not expensive. New study shows they may reduce frequency of hot flashes. Also might reduce triglycerides and help with weight loss in men on LHRH. If you have a fish allergy, you can try one of the new algae-based omega-3 supplements.

Complementary & Alternative Treatments	Advantages & Disadvantages
Flaxseed powder (2 to 3 tablespoons a day on foods or in beverages)	Cheap, high in fiber and omega-3 fatty acids, heart healthy, but lacks studies in men.
Magnesium supplements (250 to 600 mg/day in a clinical trial currently using magnesium oxide)	Cheap and safe. However, most of the recent minimal research has been with women suffering from hot flashes during breast cancer treatment.
Red clover pills	Moderate to expensive in price. Mixed research in men. May have side effects, and results are similar to a placebo.
Soy products/protein (several servings a day or 20 to 40 grams of soy protein per day)	Cheap. Natural products (beans, powder, tofu) are heart healthy and may be more effective and healthy as compared to soy pills. As dosage is increased, so do gastrointestinal side effects.

Prescriptions and Medical Procedures

These options are more effective than lifestyle and complementary options in dealing with moderate to severe hot flashes. However, they can be expensive, and all of them have side effects. If using them, always be sure to ask for generic equivalents to reduce your overall cost. On average, these treatments should reduce hot flash symptoms from 50 to 75 percent for severe sufferers.

Prescription Drugs	Advantages & Disadvantages
Clonidine pills or patches (0.05 mg twice a day or 0.1 mg once a day)	Least effective, but usually cheap in price.
Cyproterone acetate (100 mg daily)	Steroidal anti-androgens that are not available in some countries, including the U.S. Very effective (they act like progesterone), but cyproterone may have cardiovascular risks

Prescription Drugs	Advantages & Disadvantages
Estrogen pills, patches, and injections(multiple dose options, usually less than 1 mg)	Very effective, usually cheap, and they reduce bone loss. However, some forms have serious cardiovascular and other potential risks (can cause blood clots, breast enlargement).
Gabapentin pills (average dose is 300 mg three times a day) or Pregabalin pills (average dose is 75 mg twice daily)	Very effective, have a range of doses, but can cause drowsiness and dizziness.
Progesterone pills, injections (megesterol acetate at 20 to 40 mg a day, or medroxyprogesterone acetate at 20 mg a day, or intramuscular injection of 150–400 mg total of medroxyprogesterone acetate as needed)	Most effective, but may increase weight gain, reduce HDL (good cholesterol), and libido (sex drive).
SSRIs & SNRIs pills Citalopram Desvenlafaxine Fluoxetine Paroxetine Sertraline Venlafaxine (multiple doses available, but 75 mg a day of venlafaxine is one of the most popular)	Moderately to very effective, but has gastrointestinal (constipation) and sexual side effects. May cause weight gain, and some have cardiovascular issues. Recent large clinical trial showed that progesterone agents work better and seem to be safer. However, these medications may be more effective for men undergoing cancer treatments with depression issues.

INCONTINENCE

Also known as loss of urinary control.

What is it? Why does it happen? Incontinence is a partial or complete loss of urinary control. Treatments for prostate cancer such as surgery, radiation, and cryosurgery are the more common causes, but this side effect has been reduced dramatically over the years. Today, only a small percentage of patients experience incontinence that requires a pad after treatment. What are the signs or symptoms? Simply, patients may have the inability to control urine flow, resulting in leaking or dribbling.

Prevention and Treatment Options

Lifestyle and Diet Tips

The prevention and treatment of incontinence is a large field of medicine and is beyond the scope of this book. You should consult with a urologist if faced with a problem in this area. However, there are many options available for prevention and treatment, including Kegel exercises (also called special perineal exercises) that can be done before and after treatment. These exercises involve strengthening the pelvic muscles by deliberately stopping and starting the urine flow. When not urinating, the same results can be achieved by tightening the muscles of the pelvis or buttocks. Regular practice of the Kegel exercises (talk to your doctor about how often) may reduce leakage or correct it permanently according to some doctors, but the results may vary from individual to individual. These exercises are generally repeated at least several times a day for several weeks or months.

Keep in mind that special undergarments, briefs, pads, pills, inserts (catheter), injections, biofeedback, acupuncture, melatonin, many prescription agents, and even surgery are all viable treatment options for mild to severe incontinence.

INSOMNIA

What is it? Why does it happen? This side effect, caused by cancer treatment or by the stress and anxiety of day-to-day life, is arguably the one that receives the least attention (along with stress itself). Despite the large variety of the possible reasons for this, it is important to resolve the problem because a lack of sleep increases the risk of experiencing all sorts of other issues—fatigue, depression, anxiety, stress. What are the signs or symptoms? Cancer patients tend to get a lot of information on fatigue and advice to improve energy levels and stay alert, but often little is said about sleeplessness.

Some individuals simply toss and turn the majority of the night and do not wake up rested because of a lack of sleep. Since sleep is crucial to physical and mental health, when someone does not get enough sleep the result is a variety of daytime symptoms, such as memory and concentration issues, irritability, fatigue, immune problems, and an increased risk of accidents.

It is important to consider what part of your sleep pattern has changed, and to describe this accurately to your doctor. For example, is there any problem in staying asleep (sleep maintenance), or just falling asleep (sleep induction), or both? What do you think is the reason for your lack of sleep? Have you tried any sleep remedies? Which ones and were they effective? Insomnia is more complex than it sounds. There are many reasons why people have trouble sleeping, and proper identification of the problem will help in finding a solution.

Prevention and Treatment Options

Lifestyle and Diet Tips

- Regular exercise before dinnertime can help to reduce stress and relax your body.
- Avoid tobacco products and secondhand smoke. Chemicals from the smoke have a stimulating effect on the body.
- Alcohol increases the chances that you will fall asleep (sleep induction), but it also reduces the chances that you will experience deep and refreshing sleep. Therefore, alcohol is not a good way to help you sleep. Alcohol also makes you get up at night to use the bathroom, another way that it interrupts deep sleep.
- Caffeine in the evening works as a stimulant to keep you awake because its half-life (a measure of how long it stays in large amounts in the body) is approximately 5 hours. Consuming caffeine after 5 p.m. increases the chances of insomnia.
- Hot shower? Not quite! Cold shower—yes! In reality, some people get better sleep after a hot shower because they get cold coming out of the shower or bath. Research shows that, as your sleep center in your brain cools down

slightly, it is easier for a person to fall asleep. So, the bedroom should be at a slightly cooler temperature and shielded from sunlight.

- Bright lights or alarm clocks, computer screens, and televisions should not be in the bedroom because they can make it difficult to sleep.
- Sleep to get rest. However, oversleeping can make it difficult to sleep the next night. Setting an alarm to wake youself every morning at a consistent time, including on weekends, is a good idea. Also, avoid long naps during the day. Limit yourself to a refreshing 20- or 30-minute rest during the daytime.
- Try only to go to bed when you are sleepy, because attempting to force yourself to sleep can increase the number of sleepless nights.
- A sleep study is an excellent way to see how you really sleep. In a perfect world, everyone would have a one-night sleep study. A study monitors your sleep either in a clinical environment or at home using a measuring device. Sleep studies have worked miracles for some individuals by diagnosing all sorts of things, such as sleep apnea (interruptions in breathing during sleep). Diagnosis may lead to finding appropriate methods to correct the underlying problem interrupting sleep.
- Research has found that numerous foods not only contain tryptophan (the amino acid that can be converted to melatonin in the body to help you sleep), but also melatonin itself. Oats, sweet corn, rice, bananas, barley, cherries, ginger and even tomatoes contain melatonin, and egg whites, spirulina, and animal meats contain tryptophan. However, it is questionable whether the amounts of tryptophan and melatonin in most foods help to promote sleep. On the other hand, high-carbohydrate meals such as pasta, breads, and dairy products can make you feel full and make you sleepy.

Dietary Supplements and Over-the-Counter Options

- Decongestants and some other over-the-counter

medications have stimulant properties, so read your labels. They can keep you up, so try and take them early in the day if you need to use them.

- Antihistamine compounds, such as diphenhydramine (Benadryl), can be found in many cold and allergy medications. They are also used in many over-the-counter sleep aids because these ingredients can easily make you sleepy. However, they may also affect your thinking and balance and cause dry eyes and mouth and urinary problems. They should not be used over the long term but rather for a few days, if needed. Also, although antihistamines can cause drowsiness, they do not help to promote deep sleep or improve sleep overall—another reason they should not be used for long periods of time.
- As we discussed earlier, melatonin is a sleep inducer, which means it helps you fall asleep, but not necessarily stay asleep. In addition to food sources, melatonin can be taken in a supplement at 0.5–1 mg on average 15–30 minutes before sleeping. Many individuals are recommended 3 to 5 mg a day of melatonin or more, but keep in mind that physiologic doses of melatonin are only 0.5 to 1 mg per day. In other words, the amount of melatonin that is needed to get you to sleep is much lower than what is usually recommended. Additionally, taking too much melatonin can make you tired the next day. Melatonin can potentially be combined with some prescription drug sleep aids, but talk to your doctor first.
- Valerian (also known as Valeriana officinalis) is actually the dietary supplement that has occasionally been effective at helping someone fall asleep and stay in deeper and more refreshing states of sleep. Never combine this supplement with other sleeping pills or other central nervous system depressants, such as strong pain medications. Be sure to discuss with your health care professional to see if this supplement makes sense for your situation and if there are other specific drug interactions that may be of concern. Some clinical trials have reported diarrhea as a

potential side effect in a small percentage of patients. Valerian should be purchased as a root extract with at least 0.8% valerenic acids in it (this is the active ingredient). It may take several weeks to become effective. Studies that have used 200 to 600 mg (most common is arguably 600 mg) of valerian daily have shown dosages in this range to be the safest and most effective usage. The supplement is usually taken 30 to 60 minutes before bedtime. Most studies involved using valerian by itself and not mixed in with other herbs, so this would seem advisable for patients as well.

- Other herbal sleep supplements are not worth your money because there are so many good prescription sleep aids. Passionflower, hops, wild lettuce, Jamaica dogwood, and others might sound interesting, but save your money because there isn't research to support their use for insomnia. Behavioral therapy or sleep hygiene advice can be provided by a sleep expert.

Prescriptions and Medical Procedures

- Diuretic drugs can disturb sleep, so try to take these pills early in the day.
- There are a number of very effective prescription options, so discuss the possibilities with your doctor. Keep in mind that they tend to work quickly so most of them should be taken just before going to bed. Some of the more common prescription medications are nonbenzodiazepine sedatives, such as Ambien (zolpidem), Lunesta (eszopiclone), and Sonata (zaleplon).
- Rozerem (ramelteon) is actually a prescription drug that stimulates the melatonin receptors in the brain to act as though they are receiving a more potent version of melatonin. It is approved for individuals who have difficulty falling asleep.
- Benzodiazepine sedatives include Ativan (lorazepam), Clonazepam (klonopin), Dalmane (flurazepam), Eurodin/Prosom (estazolam), Halcion (triazolam), and Restoril (temazepam).

- Some antidepressants and anti-stress medications have been given to some individuals with co-existing issues (depression, stress, and sleep issues). For example, the benzodiazepine sedatives listed above are also used for stress and can help relax you.

JOINT AND MUSCLE PAIN

Also known as arthralgia and myalgia.

What is it? Why does it happen? Joint and muscle pain are not uncommon side effects of cancer treatments. Some cases are probably due to the everyday aches and pains that individuals can experience, but there are also a large number of individuals who experience them for the first time or find that their situation worsens during cancer treatment. Researchers are not exactly sure why it happens, but perhaps we can learn something from breast cancer treatment. One of the most powerful and effective drugs (an aromatase inhibitor) used to treat breast cancer dramatically lowers the levels of female hormone in the body, and a fairly widespread side effect when taking the drug is joint pain. It may be true that male and female hormones protect the joints in some way so that, when men have their testosterone levels reduced by prostate cancer treatment, they also experience aches and pains in some areas of the body. Regardless of the reason, there are many simple treatments for this condition listed in this section.

What are the signs or symptoms? The joints and muscles can become sore to very sore and even stiff in some cases. It can be difficult to carry out daily activities or to sleep. Joint pain or soreness may occur at several locations in the body at once or be isolated in one place. There can also be swelling and even redness in the area, and it may be sensitive to the touch. Elbow, hip, knee, ankle, shoulder, and neck joints, and even the tiny joints in the hands and feet can be sites of discomfort. Do note that it is critical to determine with your doctor whether the discomfort is coming from a joint, a muscle, both, or from another place entirely, such as a bone or nerve

Prevention and Treatment Options

Lifestyle and Diet Tips

- Heating pad and/or ice, applied several times during the day or at night, can help.
- Apply heat to a specific troublesome joint before physical activity, and use a cold pack after exercise.
- Electrolyte-based sports drinks have potassium, magnesium, and even some sugar and caffeine that may help with muscle soreness and, in some cases, joint pain. In fact, try coconut water, which has more potassium than a banana.
- Losing just a little weight can take pressure off some joints and reduce pain.
- Taking an Epsom salt bath makes sense. You can purchase cheap magnesium sulfate (Epsom salt) at a pharmacy and pour the recommended amount into a hot bath. This can be very effective when used regularly to reduce the ache of joint or muscle pain. Magnesium is able to penetrate into the skin and provides an anti-inflammatory or pain-relieving effect along with the hot bath. Epsom salts are both a cheap and an effective remedy. Just make sure that the hot bath water and salt is completely covering the affected area for at least 10–15 minutes.
- Gelatin (yes, that stuff at the grocery store) is a home remedy for joint pain that is very popular and safe, but needs some research. There have been so many individuals that claim benefits that it is difficult to ignore. Besides, it actually makes sense that it might work! Gelatin is a protein that comes from the collagen inside an animal's (cattle, pigs, and horses) skin and bones. When consumed, it may reach the joint and provide some protection or lubrication. Gelatin substitutes are also available that have similar gel forming features and may also lubricate the joints. For example, liquid fruit pectin or konjak (another gelatinous fiber) are options. They can be combined with

a low-calorie liquid or taken as a pill. Some think all this gelatin pain relief is nothing more than a placebo effect, but that is not what recent evidence suggests. It is a very safe option, so why not try it?

- Magnet therapy is backed by little evidence that it works. It isn't recommended if it will be costly.

Dietary Supplements and Over-the-Counter Options

The many dietary supplements for joint and muscle issues listed here may be surprising to some readers. Prescription pain killers get a good deal of attention, but these supplements often fail to get their due credit. While they may not be as effective as the pain killers, they have had minimal safety issues thus far, so they merit consideration. If you want to consider taking any of the options, please be sure to discuss them with your doctor first. She or he can help determine if they fit your situation. Some are available in pill, liquid, and patch options, so be sure to check for your preference.

- Over-the-counter pain relievers are options for both muscle and joint pain, but remember that ibuprofen (Advil, Motrin, and others) can cause ulcer and blood pressure issues. While acetaminophen (Tylenol) does not involve these issues, it can increase liver toxicity when combined with alcohol on a regular basis.
- Vitamin D supplements taken to normalize blood levels (30–40 ng/ml) have been known to provide both muscle and joint pain relief for some patients. Vitamin D receptors are found on muscle tissue, and this inexpensive method is worth a try for some patients.
- Fish oil (1000–2000 mg per day of the active ingredients EPA and DHA) has been supported by good evidence recently that it may reduce aches and pains in the back, knee, hip, and other joints. Fish oil works as a natural anti-inflammatory. Note: Keep in mind that just because a fish oil pill claims 1000 to 1500 mg per softgel or capsule does *not* mean it contains that amount of the active ingredients EPA and DHA. You need to examine the label closely to note the actual amount of EPA and DHA or

omega-3 compounds in the capsule. For example, a popular fish oil brand advertises that each softgel contains around 1400 mg, but when you look on the back of the ingredients it shows that about 950 mg of that has omega-3 compounds (EPA and DHA). Fish oil is available in pills or liquid. Always keep in mind that as the dosage of fish oil increases, so does the chance that it may act as a blood thinner. Talk with your doctor, especially if you are already on a blood thinner.

- Glucosamine is a hexosamine sugar (amino acid sugar). It is a basic building block for the production of glycosaminoglycans (GAGs) and proteoglycans, which are important components of articular cartilage. It is naturally produced by the body and widely distributed in connective tissue, including cartilage. Glucosamine supplements come in pills and liquid form and are generally derived from crab shells or corn. Doses of 500 to 1500 mg per day of glucosamine sulfate taken over several weeks may be associated with a reduction in joint pain and an improvement in function versus a placebo. The potential side effects of glucosamine are unknown at this time, but individuals have reported blood thinning, stomach upset, and excess gas in some cases.
- Chondroitin sulfate is a glycosaminoglycan found in proteoglycans of articular cartilage. It is a complex carbohydrate molecule that helps retain water in cartilage. It generally comes from shark, pig, or cow cartilage. It may increase proteoglycan synthesis in the chondrocytes of articular cartilage. Doses of 500 to 1200 mg a day have provided relief by themselves or when combined with glucosamine.
- S-adenosylmethionine (SAM-e) is a nutritional supplement that has received a lot of attention recently in the United States. It is widely used in Europe for a variety of conditions, including osteoarthritis and depression. A review of numerous clinical trials of SAM-e as compared to a placebo or NSAIDs concluded that the existing evidence points toward at least an equal efficacy of

this supplement for osteoarthritis. More clinical studies are needed. Dosages in the studies ranged from 600 to 1200 mg per day for at least 30 to 90 days. More safety data are needed with these supplements, and they are not inexpensive (as is the case with glucosamine). In the meantime, the butanedisulfonate salt form of SAM-e is generally recommended because it may have the best stability and is absorbed by your body at the highest rate. However, if you cannot locate this form, the others should also be helpful.

- Pycnogenol comes from French maritime pine bark extract. In two recent clinical trials, it helped to reduce joint pain and stiffness (from osteoarthritis) by 35 to 55 percent, allowing patients to cut back on their pain medications. The most effective daily dose on average was 50 mg twice a day, taken after meals (breakfast and dinner). One drawback is that it can be expensive.
- Methylsulfonylmethane (MSM) is a compound that has natural sulfur in it. It is claimed that it finds its way into or near joint tissue to relieve discomfort. A few small studies using 1000 to 3000 mg a day have demonstrated some small benefit. Perhaps taking this compound in the same pill or liquid as a glucosamine chondroitin product offers the best chance for some success with minimal harm.
- Over the counter pain-relief creams, gels, or patches such as capsaicin (an ingredient from the pepper plant), seem to work better for the hand, knee, and shoulder, and not as well on the hip because this joint is deeper in the body. However, be careful and apply the product using gloves or a cotton swab. If you get capsaicin on your fingers and into your eye, the burning sensation can be quite painful and potentially harmful.
- Newer and probably less effective creams, such as hyaluronic acid (HA), for joint pain now exist. In addition, hyaluronic acid dietary supplements are also available. The research on the pill is sparse compared to the research on topical cream. However, the overall research on both is minimal.

- Other new joint creams and pills contain cetylated fatty acids, which are simply naturally occurring fats. These creams and pills are backed by some minimal clinical research, and one ingredient, cetyl myristoleate, is the focus of the most research right now and probably acts as a joint lubricant.
- DMSO (dimethyl sufoxide) is a sulfur-containing compound from wood pulp. It comes in a gel, liquid, or roll-on, and can be applied to the area of joint pain. Some people have developed an allergic rash and itching reaction to this product.
- Be careful about over-the-counter pain relief creams that contain aspirin. These creams can be absorbed into the blood stream and work as a blood thinner. Your doctor may be concerned with that side effect of the cream so be sure to check with her or him before using them.
- Vitamin C is involved in maintaining the strength of bones and joints as we get older. Recently there have been several large preliminary studies that suggest that getting vitamin C from supplements and food may slightly reduce the risk of bone loss and joint pain. It may be worth trying 500 to 1000 mg daily since vitamin C has been shown to be a very safe dietary supplement in standard dosages.
- Eggshell protein or eggshell membrane is a new supplement backed by preliminary research that suggests it may help with joint pain. There are egg protein powders that are wonderful sources of protein when a scoop is mixed with water. Your local health food store should carry these newer options, which may be worth considering.
- Avocado/soybean unsaponifiable supplements now have several clinical studies to suggest that they may help with joint issues, especially in the knee and hip. The supplements are actually an extract from avocados and soybeans that appear to reduce inflammation and stimulate some repair. In some countries the combination is actually an approved

prescription medication, but more research is needed. The suggested dose from the studies is around 300 mg per day. Apparently trying to consume this amount from avocados or soybeans themselves is virtually impossible because only 1 percent of the oil (the unsaponifiable portion) seems to carry the joint activity. That said, saturated oils, such as avocado and soybean, contain omega fatty acids that can be beneficial for the joints in theory. Consuming more avocados or using a teaspoon of soybean oil a day is certainly worth a try.

- Another interesting supplement is turmeric (the popular spice used in curry powders). It has demonstrated some anti-inflammatory effects in preliminary studies in rheumatoid arthritis, but it has not been well tested for joint pain. Safe to say that the jury is still out.
- Acupuncture is backed by some evidence that it helps to alleviate joint pain, but this is a preliminary finding from some smaller studies. It can be costly, but may be worth trying, as it doesn't have the potential for interaction with other treatments.
- Low-level laser therapy for joint pain sounds a bit far-fetched, but there is some minimal research to suggest that receiving this type of treatment regularly may provide some pain relief. The cost may be the biggest issue, and finding a qualified health care professional who offers this treatment on a regular basis is not easy. Several treatments can cost hundreds of dollars, so this may be an option to consider only if other treatments are not working. Applying low-level laser energy to an area may stimulate a repair response by the body or may simply reduce inflammation in the area. A recent medical article suggesting that lasers may improve neck pain has renewed interest in this area.
- Quinine is popular for muscle cramps (not joint pain) as long as it is consumed in moderation from tonic water, but the side effects of more concentrated sources of quinine, for example a pill, could be very toxic.

Prescriptions and Medical Procedures

- Steroid pills have been used in some patients who experience more extreme muscle and joint pain. In rare cases when muscle pain has been felt from head to toe, prescription steroids have provided wonderful relief. Steroid injections have also provided temporary relief in specific joint areas that hurt.
- Prescription painkillers are discussed in more depth in the pain section, but they are always effective options that come with catches. For example, Celebrex works well, but has an increased risk of cardiovascular disease.
- Lovaza is a prescription fish oil pill that is highly concentrated and contains almost 1000 mg per pill of the active ingredients in fish oil (EPA and DHA). Newer over-the-counter bottled liquid fish oil, and even the softgels, are now available and compete with this prescription. In many cases, the nonprescription options may cost a lot less. Therefore, the prescription fish oil is not worth it for most individuals unless your insurance plan almost completely covers it, making it cost less than the over-the-counter options.

MOUTH AND CANKER SORES

Also known as stomatitis or oral mucositis.

What is it? Why does it happen? Mouth sores can occur within one week following an infusion of Taxotere chemotherapy and other cancer drugs. Some types of chemotherapy work by blocking the replication of rapidly dividing abnormal or cancer cells, but also can impact normal cells that are dividing rapidly. This is known to affect bone, gastrointestinal tract, and hair cells, but less attention is paid to the mouth. Cells in the mouth also replicate at a rapid rate, and it is not uncommon to have mouth sores and pain during the chemotherapy. Mucositis refers to problems ranging from the mouth, to the stomach, to the intestines, and down to the anal area that can occur from cancer treatment. Oral mucositis or stomatitis just means that the problem is located in the mouth.

Canker sores are small mouth ulcers or lesions and are common in patients with and without cancer. There are a number of reasons they occur, including immune changes and stress, and they can be caused in some patients by consuming acidic foods. Even a rough tooth surface or dental appliance can cause canker sores. Canker sores are generally mildly annoying as opposed to mouth sores that can be more troublesome for cancer patients. Patients can generally obtain relief using the over-the-counter methods below.

What are the signs and symptoms? Oral mucositis usually starts as a burning sensation somewhere in the mouth. Areas can appear red and inflamed, and the area(s) can become more eroded until eventually sores (ulcerations) appear. There may be some discomfort and pain associated with these mouth and/or tongue sores. The lips can also appear dry and irritated in this situation. It can take several weeks following chemotherapy for the sore areas to heal.

The following World Health Organization (WHO) scale is one of many used to classify the severity of stomatitis.

Grade 1 = Redness and soreness
Grade 2 = Ulcers, but able to eat solid foods
Grade 3 = Ulcers, and can only consume a liquid diet because of the stomatitis
Grade 4 = Ulcers, and cannot consume foods and beverages because of the stomatitis

The following recommendations to prevent and treat stomatitis or mouth sores come from either chemotherapy or head and neck radiation studies; both treatments can cause stomatitis. Because stomatitis pain is one of the more common problems with this side effect, pain control is a very important, if not the most important, first step in treating this condition. In general, these preventive and treatment steps should be kept in mind to reduce the risk of stomatitis and the severity of this side effect:

- Pain control
- Maintaining good nutrition

- Good oral hygiene to prevent infection
- Reducing dry mouth (which makes infection worse and more likely)
- Management of any bleeding in the mouth

Prevention and Treatment Options

Lifestyle and Diet Tips

- Eat foods that are at room temperature or even cold, avoiding foods that may be too warm.
- Eat soft or semi-liquid foods that are soothing and easy to swallow, such as macaroni and cheese, soft ice cream, soups, milk shakes, mashed potatoes, scrambled eggs, or even baby food. A blender or food processor can be used to puree cooked foods. Most foods can be cut, mashed, or simply chopped into very tiny pieces, such as tuna in a can, fruits, and vegetables. Talk to a cancer nutritionist to get a better idea about nutritional support if you have stomatitis.
- Avoid acidic or irritating beverages or foods, such as citrus juices, tomato juice, spicy and overly salty foods, or even rough foods, such as popcorn, granola, toast, raw vegetables, or hard tree nuts.
- Alcohol or tobacco can make the problem more painful and increase the healing time.
- Use a straw for any liquid, especially if you have numerous sores that make it difficult to use a cup or container to consume liquids.
- When possible, keep dry foods moist by using butter, margarine, butter substitutes, gravy, and sauces.
- Use lip balm or petroleum jelly for dry lips.
- Before brushing your teeth, select an extra soft tooth brush and soak the toothbrush in some warm water so that the bristles are as soft as possible going into your mouth. Rinse with warm salt water or sterile water after meals and at bedtime. Also, be sure to rinse the toothbrush well and place it in a dry place. Flossing daily and/or using a Water-Pik is critical to improve oral hygiene and reduce the risk of this problem. Good oral hygiene not only prevents an infection in the mouth

or helps keep an existing infection from getting worse, but it may also prevent an infection in the mouth from spreading into the rest of the body.

- Do not use mouthwashes with alcohol in them, for these can be painful. Ask your doctor or pharmacist for a mild mouthwash, for example one that contains baking soda. Another option is to make your own mouthwash using salt and baking soda by mixing one teaspoon of each per unit of water. Baking soda works as a cleansing agent by loosening debris and dissolving mucus. The combination of salt and baking soda increases the pH of the mouth (makes it more basic) and prevents the overgrowth of bacteria that thrive in an acidic environment. As an alternative, you can purchase a saline solution at a pharmacy. Saline mouthwashes are also believed to increase tissue repair and healing. Swish and spit multiple times a day (up to 6 times) for relief.
- Povidone-iodine is another popular antiseptic agent that seems to be effective against oral bacteria. In one randomized trial, it appeared to be effective at reducing stomatitis from radiation when used as highly diluted (1:8) mouthwash. If you want to consider using it for chemotherapy-induced stomatitis, please talk to your doctor. It is important not to swallow iodine, as it is toxic. Generally speaking, mouthwashes can be used at any time to prevent or treat stomatitis.
- "Oral cooling" (cryotherapy) of the mouth by sucking on ice chips or crushed ice causes blood vessels in the area to constrict and reduces blood flow to the area. Thus, it was thought that doing this several times a day could limit drug delivery to the cells of the mouth. Additionally, two randomized studies have shown that it may be effective at preventing stomatitis. Definitely an easy and safe method to try.
- Honey has been getting a lot of attention lately as a natural anti-microbial product and a substance that promotes wound healing. Honey has a variety of

compounds that do seem potentially to be effective for a variety of conditions. A few small studies have used honey several times a day on mouth sores to promote healing, and there is some suggestion that it seems to help, and may prevent, infections in the area. However, other unique natural mouthwashes such as aloe vera and chamomile have not been effective.

- Anesthetic rub-on gels, such as Orajel, can help reduce the discomfort, and pain medications such as ibuprofen, Motrin, naproxen, and others can help.
- Dry mouth (xerostomia), with or without stomatitis, is a problem because it makes it difficult to eat and increases the risk of pain and infection (saliva has anti-microbial properties). Chew sugarless gum if there is a need to stimulate some extra saliva due to dry mouth. A simple solution, sipping water, may help. Saliva substitutes can be purchased. Also, ask your doctor about medications known as cholinergic agents, which can help if the other methods for dry mouth are not sufficient. Cholinergic drugs can improve salivary flow but also come with a number of potential side effects. Interestingly, there have been several preliminary studies of acupuncture that has shown a benefit for patients with chronic dry mouth.

Dietary Supplements and Over-the-Counter Options

- Avoid irritating the situation with acidic dietary supplements, particularly ascorbic acid or plain vitamin C. If you take vitamin C, it is available on the market in plenty of non-acidic or buffered options. Look for the words "calcium ascorbate" on the ingredients list; this is one of the most-researched non-acidic forms of vitamin C.
- Traumeel S is a homeopathic medication that has 12 botanical compounds and 2 minerals. It has been around for over 50 years, and it has been proposed to help a variety of conditions. When used as a mouth wash in a randomized and placebo-controlled study, it significantly reduced the severity and duration of oral mucositis from chemotherapy.

- L-glutamine is a compound and an amino acid dietary supplement used for the support and maintenance of intestinal growth and function, and there are large reductions in the compound during some cancer treatments. However, as a preventive therapy for stomatitis, it has not been very effective overall when swallowed as a dietary supplement. There is research ongoing using the compound in a homemade mouthwash preparation to determine whether it can promote healing. For that reason, it might be worth a try when mixed with baking soda and salt in a mouthwash.
- Some preliminary results suggest that zinc sulphate (50 mg of elemental zinc) taken 3 times a day might lessen the severity of stomatitis. In low doses, zinc is backed by plenty of research to suggest that it can help with tissue repair. However, at higher doses you need to be careful; gastrointestinal problems, such as diarrhea, can occur. Zinc gluconate is another form of zinc that is more easily absorbed and has had fewer side effects in clinical trials outside of cancer, so perhaps a low-dose zinc gluconate tablet would make more sense. This form of zinc has been the one primarily used in cold lozenges for kids. Doses of 30 to 45 mg a day of this form of zinc have been shown to be safe in adults, but its impact on stomatitis is unknown at this time.
- Melatonin has some preliminary laboratory research showing that it may reduce dry mouth and provide some protection against mouth sores. If you are using 0.5 to 1 mg of melatonin to help you sleep, then you might receive a 2-for-1 benefit with mouth sore reduction. Otherwise, its usefulness on mouth sores and dry mouth is unclear at this time.
- Patients with extensive canker sores may benefit from taking 1000 mcg daily of vitamin B12. A recent study of patients taking the supplement for 6 months showed a reduction in the number of canker sores, the duration of the sores, and in the level of pain they caused. Other dietary

supplements reporting some success on canker sores are buffered (non-acidic) vitamin C (1000 to 2000 mg/day), brewer's yeast (500 mg/day), and bee propolis (500 mg/day). You should discuss possible supplements with your doctor if your canker sores are severe.

Prescriptions and Medical Procedures

There are a variety of prescription mouthwashes, pills, and other agents that your doctor can use, including growth factors (usually used in some other cancers), anti-inflammatories and pain medications, antioxidants, lasers, and anti-infective medications. The following is just a quick review of some of the more common prescriptions that you should discuss with you doctor.

- Topical anesthetic agents and pain pills or liquids. Talk to your doctor about pain control pills and/or pain control mouthwashes, such as 2% viscous lidocaine that can be mixed with a variety of substances including diphenhydramine and a soothing covering agent such as Maalox or Kaopectate. These mixtures or agents can provide short-term pain relief. Also, keep in mind that if there is any bleeding, the doctor can talk to you about using a topical clotting agent (apply it right on the source of bleeding), such as a fibrin glue or gelatin sponge.
- Chlorhexidine (concentrations of at least 0.12%) mouthwashes are still popular but have only been minimally effective against stomatitis. As a preventive mouthwash used several times a day, it has minimal effects. However, benzydamine hydrochloride is a non-steroidal anti-inflammatory mouthwash that also is supported by minimal positive research in the area of chemotherapy-induced stomatitis. Talk to your doctor about the latest research on this and other mouth washes.
- Sucralfate (Carafate) is a mouthwash or a protective prescription product that forms an adhesive paste-like substance that attaches to areas that are damaged. It is known as a "mouth-coating" agent. The protective coating provides a continuous barrier to further potential irritation

and damage. This protective layer also probably prevents bacteria and other microorganisms from causing an infection. These mouthwashes are used multiple times throughout the day (up to 6 times a day in some studies). However, recent analysis of a variety of studies concluded that is not very effective for preventing or treating stomatitis from radiation treatment, although it may or may not be more effective in chemotherapy.

- Your doctor may also want you to use a single or combination anti-bacterial, anti-fungal, and/or anti-viral medication to prevent or treat this problem. Bacteria, fungi, and/or a virus can cause an infection in the mouth. One example of such a combination, PTA, is a mixture of several antimicrobial agents (polymyxin E, tobramycine, and amphotericin B) that comes in a lozenge or paste and eliminates some bacteria and yeast in the mouth. It has been used to treat stomatitis or reduce its severity after radiation therapy to the head and neck, but it has not been used in preventing or treating chemotherapy-induced stomatitis. Regardless, it may be an option worth trying due to its effectiveness in other areas.
- GM-CSF or G-CSF (separate drugs) promote the movement of immune cells into the mouth to provide some protection against infection and damage. Several studies show that, when given as an injection (not as a mouthwash), it seems to not only prevent immune cell reduction (neutropenia) and fever but also stomatitis.
- Low-energy lasers applied to the area of stomatitis is backed by some preliminary evidence showing that they may promote wound healing and reduce pain and inflammation. For example, studies of low-energy helium-neon lasers have shown some benefit. However, these studies were very small, so talk to your doctor about the latest options.
- Amifostine (Ethyol) is a radical-scavenging compound that protects normal cells from treatment toxicity and has been used as a preventive agent in radiation therapy against mucositis in a variety of areas of the body with some success. It may also help to relieve dry mouth. It can be

given as an injectable medication. It has the potential to reduce blood pressure significantly, so this has to be monitored while you are receiving it. Talk to your doctor about whether or not it makes sense for you if your mouth problems are caused by chemotherapy instead of radiation.

MUSCLE LOSS AND WEAKNESS

Also known as sarcopenia.

What is it? Why does it happen? Any treatment that impacts or simply reduces male hormone levels (ADT) may cause muscle changes, ranging from muscle weakness to muscle loss and pain (see also the joint and muscle pain section).

What are the signs or symptoms? Patients may notice a reduction in muscle strength and muscle size, especially in arms, shoulders, and legs. Everyday lifting and strength activities, from working out to carrying groceries, may be noticeably more difficult.

Prevention and Treatment Options

Lifestyle and Diet Tips

No surprise here! Weightlifting or resistance exercise and regular aerobic exercise of any type are the best ways to reduce the risk of muscle loss and weakness. HRPC patients should always check with their doctors before starting or changing an exercise program because your condition may impact what types of exercises are appropriate.

Higher protein intakes may help, but talk to a nutritionist about how much you really need because extremely high protein intake can cause abnormal changes in your kidneys, especially if you already have kidney issues.

Dietary Supplements and Over-the-Counter Options

- Recent research suggests that most men on ADT do not get the recommended daily intake of calcium, which is 1200 to 1500 mg per day. That, along with vitamin D, may help this problem. Recent research with vitamin D suggests that supplementation with an average of 800 to 1000 IU may help reduce muscle atrophy and/or pain, but ideally it would be best to first get a vitamin D blood test (a 25-OH vitamin D test) before deciding with your doctor whether you need more or less.

- A common dietary supplement that is used to improve muscle size and strength is creatine monohydrate powder, but the research is preliminary on this product. Most studies use only 5 grams or a teaspoon a day in a beverage for men who lift weights on a regular basis. It may be better to take some minimal-to-moderate amino acid/whey protein powder supplementation that can be added to water. It should contain around 100 calories per 8 ounces (around 20 grams of high-quality protein per serving). Recent research suggests this may work with weightlifting to reduce muscle loss and even help with weight loss at just 1 or 2 servings per day. As always, talk to your doctor about the latest research.

Prescriptions and Medical Procedures

Some men inquire about growth hormone (GH) or other anabolic steroids to improve muscle mass, but there is a concern about long-term safety, cost, and the potentially lower quality of the muscle increase, despite a potential quantity increase. Most of these compounds should be avoided. Over-the-counter pain medications can reduce muscle and joint pain discomfort when taken on a regular basis. Rarely, some men have had generalized body aches and pain (some call it "androgen deprivation syndrome"), and doctors have been able to control this problem with the use of low-dose prescription steroid medications.

NAIL CHANGES

What is it? Why does it happen? Nails of the hands and/or feet can become discolored and painful due to the damaging effects of chemotherapy (Taxotere). The drug probably accumulates over time in the fingers and toes because there is a lowered blood supply to these areas to remove the drug. This side effect occurs in about 30 to 40 percent of patients, but it rarely cause serious problems. It is more likely to occur the longer a person is on chemotherapy.

What are the signs and symptoms? Changes in your finger and toe nails can include any of the following: some discoloration, brittleness, cessation of nail growth, bleeding underneath the nail, detachment of the nail and subsequent loss, and an infection around the nail caused by bacteria or fungi that can cause swelling, redness, or pain near the area (paronychia). Changes in the nail can cause anxiety and stress for some individuals, particularly in the case of the hand, because it may be unsightly. However, multiple prevention and treatment strategies are available.

The severity of the nail changes really depends on the number of treatments an individual has received and the total dose of drug received (more treatments means higher risk). Minimal relief generally occurs between treatment periods. The good news is that when treatment is over, the problem goes away with new nail growth (in approximately 6 months for fingernails and 12 months for toe nails).

Prevention and Treatment Options

Lifestyle and Diet Tips

- Protect the nails from dirt to help avoid infection.
- Wear comfortable shoes to avoid nail pain.
- Use nail polish and hardener to combat brittle nails or unsightly-looking nails. Try to reduce your use of nail polish removers (or use non-acetone-based remover) and false/fake nails because they can trap bacteria in the nail bed.
- Do not bite nails or cuticles.
- Clip nails short with a clean pair of nail scissors and avoid peeling or pulling off loose cuticles.
- Use cuticle cream into the cuticle area daily to help prevent dryness, splitting, and hangnails.
- Wear gloves to protect your nails when doing housework (washing dishes, gardening, etc.)

Dietary Supplements and Over-the-Counter Options

- One option is the use of frozen gloves (hypothermia gloves/mitts) or frozen slippers (hypothermia slippers). They work to prevent nail changes by reducing blood flow and delivery of the drug to the hands and feet. In order to reduce the chance of excessive cold against the skin, patients should wear a protective layer between the skin and the cold surface.

Patients who are sensitive to cold temperatures (Raynaud's syndrome, blood flow issues, or metastatic disease in these areas) should not try this therapy. One clinical trial of Taxotere published in 2005 found that the Elasto-Gel flexible glove (Southwest Technologies, Inc., www.elastogel.com or www.buyelastogel.com) was potentially helpful. This glove covers the hand similar to a mitten (fingers together and thumb separate). The gloves were frozen for at least 3 hours at about -25 to -30 degrees Celsius (about -13 to -22 degrees Farenheit). Glycerin in the glove helps to maintain the cold after it is placed on the hand. Patients wore the glove for a total of 90 minutes (15 minutes before Taxotere, during the hour-long infusion, and an additional 15 minutes after the infusion). Approximately halfway through treatment, patients were fitted with a new glove so that the cold could be sustained. It was found that nail problems, including having nails fall off, were significantly fewer in the hands that were treated with the gloves as compared to non-treated hands. You should discuss this therapy with your doctor before purchasing either the gloves or slippers.

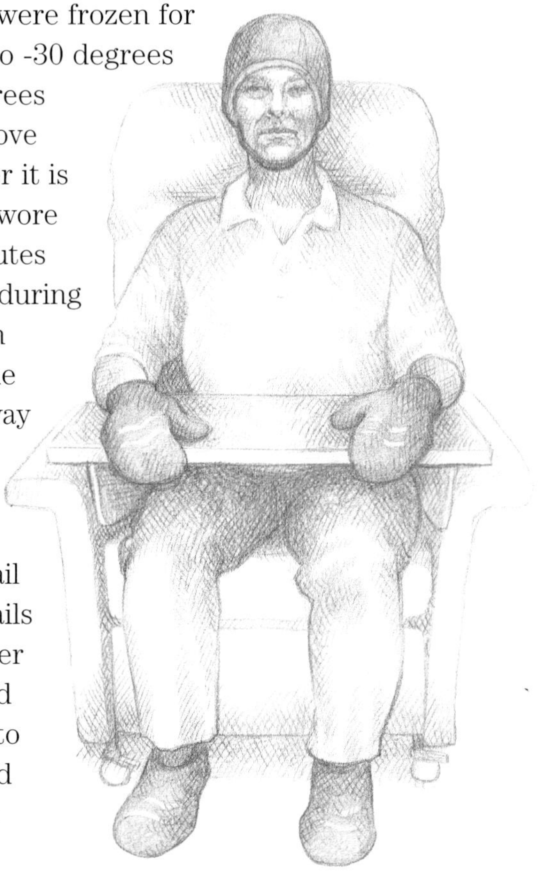

This patient is wearing a scalp cooling cap and hypothermia gloves and slippers. Used during chemotherapy treatment, the cap may reduce hair loss and the gloves and slippers may help with nail changes patients sometimes experience.

- There is some evidence to suggest that preventing and treating neuropathy (nerve changes) may reduce nail problems. In the peripheral neuropathy side effect section of this book, numerous preventive options are discussed, including the use of the dietary supplement alpha-lipoic

acid. Please review that section if you have neuropathy.
- Soaking your nails in warm to hot water 2 or 3 times a day can help reduce swelling and pain if they are infected.

Prescriptions and Medical Procedures
- GM-CSF may reduce the risk of nail problems and reduce skin problems or skin reactions. Remember, this drug is already given by some doctors to reduce the risk of infections and a low white blood cell count when the neutrophil count decreases.
- Antibiotics (oral and topical) are given if the doctor believes the nail problem is caused by a bacterial infection.
- Anti-fungal medications (oral and topical) are given if the doctor believes the nail problem is also caused by a fungal infection.
- If a nail detaches from the nail bed, there is a higher risk of infection because the protective covering has been temporarily lost. In this situation, inquire with your doctor about topical or oral medication.

NAUSEA AND VOMITING

Also known as emesis

What is it? Why does it happen? Both nausea and vomiting are potential side effects of chemotherapy, radiation, and some novel cancer therapies. There is a specific area of the brain that controls vomiting, known as the "vomiting center." Patients vomit when this center of the brain receives a signal from the brain, gastrointestinal area (stomach or intestines), or even the inner ear, which has a built-in motion detector. Chemotherapy and other medications can cause the quick release of several compounds, including serotonin, from the intestines and other locations, which acts as a signal to the vomiting center in the brain to stimulate vomiting to occur. Many of the anti-nausea medications (anti-emetics) work by making the receptors for serotonin unavailable to cause nausea and vomiting. In some cases, there are other causes, such as anxiety, that can actually cause nausea and vomiting.

What are the signs or symptoms? Nausea is the feeling of being sick to your stomach, as if you are going to throw up. Vomiting is what happens when you empty the contents of your stomach by throwing up. Nausea and vomiting can happen within days of beginning cancer treatment or even weeks into or after treatment.

Prevention and Treatment Options

Lifestyle and Diet Tips

- Try consuming the same beverages and foods as when you might have the flu—diet or regular ginger ale, soft drinks that have lost their fizz or gone flat, bland foods, sour small candy, dry crackers, pickles. Eating 5 or 6 small meals a day may make you feel better as compared to 2 or 3 large meals. Beverages and foods that are cooler in temperature should be easier to tolerate and keep down.
- Avoid spicy, fatty, fried, or very sweet foods. Cooking and freezing several simple meals that you can reheat during times of nausea is a good idea. Also, try to let someone else prepare your food or just order out when you are feeling nauseated.
- Changing the taste of or blocking the taste of certain drinks and food with another strong taste, such as lemon or another product, has been shown to be beneficial for some individuals.
- Nutritional shakes or liquid nutritional products may be easier to keep down and will help maintain good nutritional levels.
- Keep your mouth clean by brushing at least twice a day and using mouthwash because even slightly abnormal mouth smells can increase nausea.
- Wear loose-fitting clothing, and at times of nausea go without a belt to avoid pressure on your abdomen.
- Dietary protein from lean meats, fish, eggs, and beans can reduce nausea.

Dietary Supplements and Over-the-Counter Options

- A new National Cancer Institute (NCI)–sponsored study of cancer patients showed that taking 500 to 1000 mg a day of a ginger dietary supplements (equivalent to 1/4 to 1/2 teaspoon of ground ginger) along with conventional medicines for nausea and vomiting had a wonderful result. There was a significant benefit for patients who also took ginger dietary supplements with their anti-nausea drugs during the first 3 days of chemotherapy and for days after chemotherapy. The patient's treatment schedule was: ginger supplement 3 days before, receive chemo, and ginger supplement 3 days after. Patients then stop taking ginger until 3 days before next treatment cycle. It is also interesting that higher doses (2000 mg per day) did not work better than the lower doses (500 to 1000 mg) per day. Keep this in mind if you consider starting this product.

- For individuals who have trouble taking or keeping pills down, there are now purified ginger candies, gum, and other simple options at most health food stores.
- Ginger has even become a common treatment to relieve nausea and vomiting during pregnancy, and so has vitamin B6 (pyridoxine). Therefore, if ginger does not work well in your case, you may want to discuss vitamin B6 supplementation with your doctor. Most of the effective studies used approximately 25 to 40 mg of vitamin B6 (total) a day.
- Protein powder (such as whey or soy) combined with ginger may reduce the nausea even more than ginger taken alone.
- Acupuncture (traditional or electro-stimulated) is backed by very good evidence that it can help to reduce nausea and vomiting from chemotherapy.
- Acupressure wristbands or battery-operated wristbands that vibrate are newer options, providing some pressure around the wrist area that may help reduce nausea and vomiting. They can be purchased over the counter, so talk with your doctor or pharmacist about where to get them. Wristbands are worn on both forearm areas for maximum potential effectiveness. They provide "P6 acupressure," which is the point in traditional Chinese medicine where nausea is controlled.

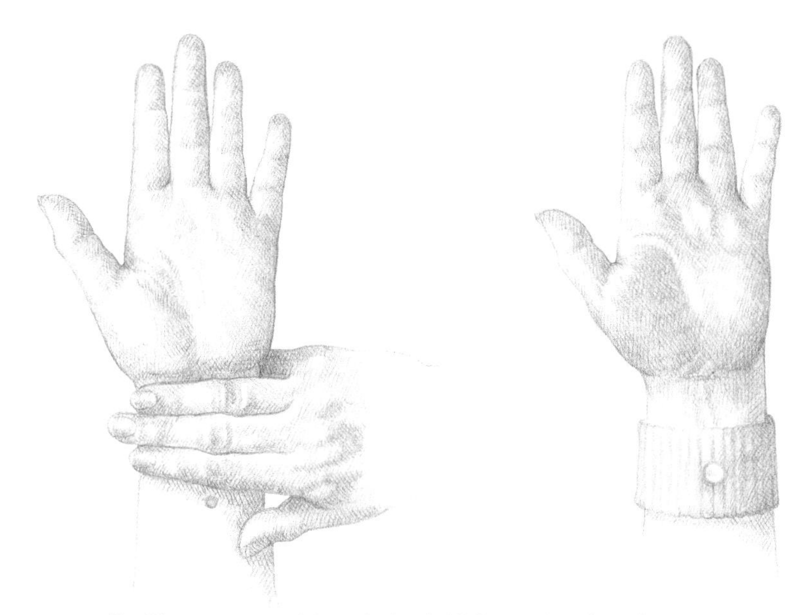

The P6 acupressure point can be located 3 fingers down from the crease of the wrist. Applying pressure here is believed to help with nausea.

Prescriptions and Medical Procedures

There are many prescription nausea and vomiting prevention and treatment drugs known collectively as antiemetics. They work by blocking the signals in the brain and intestines that cause nausea and vomiting. These medications are available in many forms today—pills, IV, and skin patches. Some examples of prescription anti-nausea agents are:

- Aloxi (palonosetron HCL)
- Anzemet (dolasetron mesylate)
- Compazine (prochlorperazine)
- Decadron (dexamethasone)
- Kytril (granisetron)
- Marinol (dronabinol)
- Tigan (trimethobenzamide)
- Torecan (triethylperazine)
- Zofran (ondansetron)

Steroids, such as dexamethasone, have the potential to prevent nausea at very low doses without suppressing the immune system or cause swelling. This is another potential benefit of getting a steroid with your cancer treatment. The drug megesterol acetate, which has been used to reduce hot flashes and stimulate appetite, has been the focus of new research suggesting it also controls nausea.

NEUROPATHY

Also known as peripheral neuropathy.

What is it? Why does it happen? Neuropathy occurs when nerves connecting the brain and the rest of the body are damaged or diseased. Damage to these nerves interrupts communication between the brain and other parts of the body and can impair muscle movement, prevent normal sensation in the arms and legs, and cause pain. Normally, you should be able to fasten your shirt buttons without difficulty or walk without looking down at your feet, but neuropathy can make this difficult.

Many things can cause neuropathy, such as injury, infection, toxic substances, a disease (diabetes is a well known cause), and chemotherapy medications such as docetaxel. This side effect increases with increasing doses and duration of chemotherapy, but it is usually mild and in most cases gets better after treatment is stopped. Research suggests that neuropathy is caused by injury or damage to the nerves and blood vessels surrounding them. Free radicals in the body produced during drug treatment do not just damage and kill cancer cells, but may also harm healthy cells and nerves.

What are the signs or symptoms? Symptoms of neuropathy usually occur in the hands and feet, but can include any of the following sensations in any area of the body:

- Burning
- Electric shock–like sensation
- Heaviness in hands and feet
- A feeling that pins and needles are touching the skin or that an area of the body is falling asleep (paresthesia)
- Itching
- Loss of reflexes (ankle and knee)
- Numbness or reduced sensation
- Prickling or stabbing feeling
- Pain

- Tingling
- Weakness

These symptoms can result in trouble walking and moving normally. They may be painful and even disabling in severe cases if not treated.

Prevention and Treatment Options

Lifestyle and Diet Tips

- Reduced cholesterol and blood pressure and maintaining a normal blood sugar may help reduce the risk of nerve damage from cardiac disease and diabetes.
- Exercise to improve muscle tone and circulation.
- Weight loss.
- Wear cotton socks to avoid blisters or sores on feet.
- Avoid crossing your legs while sitting or leaning on your elbows because this can put pressure on an already damaged nerve.
- Monitor tripping hazards.
  - Move carefully, and use handrails on stairs.
  - Wear shoes with rubber soles whenever possible.
  - Make sure rooms are well lit, without glare.
  - Create non-skid showers and bathtubs by installing bath mats.
  - Install hand rails in the bath area or use bathtub chairs for bathing.
  - Clear walkways and avoid the use of throw rugs.
- Guard against injury due to loss of sensation in fingers.
  - Be careful when grasping sharp, hot, or dangerous objects.
  - Assess your home hot water temperature to avoid burns. Be particularly careful when bathing or using hot water so skin isn't scalded.
  - Use protective gloves when washing dishes.
  - Use pot holders.

Dietary Supplements and Over-the-Counter Options

- Alpha-lipoic acid (ALA) supplements may be the only potentially effective nonprescription protective or preventive therapy (see the table following; ALA requires prescription in some countries) along with healthy changes and blood sugar control. In clinical studies, ALA is usually started at a dosage of 600 mg per day, and results are observed in as little as two weeks. Doses as high as 1800 mg per day have been used. Other dietary supplements backed by minimal research include vitamin B6, glutathione, glutamine, and N-acetylcysteine (NAC), but nothing has been shown to be as effective as ALA.

- Capsaicin cream or patches (active ingredient in hot chili peppers) can reduce neuropathic pain, so some patients may want to use it for pain that is near the surface of the skin. However, be careful and apply the product using gloves or a cotton swab. If you get capsaicin on your fingers and into your eyes, the burning sensation can be quite painful and potentially harmful.
- Vitamin E is often touted in large doses to help with neuropathy. However, the research on large doses of vitamin E and overall toxicity is enough of a concern to recommend avoidance of high doses of this supplement for any reason in cancer treatment.

Prescriptions and Medical Procedures

Following is a list of prescription medicines that may help. Alpha-lipoic acid is included here as well because it is a prescription drug in some countries. Keep in mind that if the neuropathy is so severe that it is not reduced by any method (lifestyle, supplement, drug) the physician may opt to reduce the amount of your cancer treatment drug or adjust your dosage of steroid medication. Always be sure to ask the pharmacist if generic equivalents can reduce your cost on a particular drug. While common dosages are included in the chart, your physician will determine the appropriate dosage for your situation.

Drug Name	Common Dosages	Possible Side Effects
Alpha-lipoic Acid	600–1800 mg/day	Muscle cramps, headache.
Amitriptyline	25 mg/4 times per day	Dry mouth, lightheadedness
Anticonvulsants	Multiple doses	Headache, gastrointestinal problems.
Antidepressants	Multiple doses	Gastrointestinal problems, sexual dysfunction.
Capsaicin cream (over-the-counter product)	Apply as needed	Local burning and stinging (apply with gloves).
Carbamazepine	200 mg/3 times per day	Liver toxicity, dizziness, drowsiness.
Citalopram	20 mg/2 times per day	Nausea, dizziness, headache.
Duloxetine	60 mg/2 to 4 times per day	Nausea, abnormal increase in blood sugar levels.
Gabapentin (Neurontin and generics)	600 mg/3 times per day	Dizziness, drowsiness, fluid retention (peripheral edema).
Lidoderm/Lidocaine Patches	Multiple doses	Redness and irritation at the site of the patch.
Oxycodone (OxyContin)	20 mg/2 times per day, extended release	Nausea, constipation.
Paroxetine (Paxil)	20 mg/2 times per day	Sweating, anxiety.
Phenytoin (Dilantin)	100 mg/3 times per day	Inflammation/overgrowth of gums (gingival hyperplasia).
Pregabalin (Lyrica)	150 to 300 mg/2 times day	Dizziness, sleepiness, fluid retention (peripheral edema), and mild weight gain.
Tramadol (Ultram)	50 mg/6 tabs per day	Nausea, constipation, headache, and sleepiness.
Venlafaxine (Effexor or generic)	150 mg/4 times per day, extended release	Nausea, other gastrointestinal problems including constipation, drowsiness.

NEUTROPENIA

What is it? Why does it happen? Neutropenia is a condition in which your blood has a low number of a particular type of white blood cells called neutrophils. White blood cells are the collective name for several different types of immune cells that have many roles, including fighting infection and disease. Neutrophils are one of the most important types of white blood cells because they are one of the strongest and most abundant "soldiers" in your body to help fight disease. When your neutrophil count (or total white blood cell count) decreases, there is an increased risk of infections and problems. At times, cancer treatments are stopped or delayed until blood counts return to more normal ranges.

White blood cells (and most blood cells found in the human body) are manufactured in the marrow in your bones and are released as they mature. Therefore, anything that can be slightly toxic to your bones or other body tissues can impact your blood counts. Radiation, for example, can cause a low neutrophil count in some patients. Chemotherapy, particularly Taxotere, is effective at killing cancer cells, but it can also be slightly toxic to the bone marrow. As you may recall, chemotherapy works by not allowing fast-reproducing cells of the body (healthy and unhealthy) to multiply. The fastest growing cells of the body are found in hair, the intestinal tract, and bones. With that in mind, a low neutrophil count is a logical potential side effect of chemotherapy. In fact, neutropenia is the most common blood disorder when receiving Taxotere and numerous other chemotherapy medicines, affecting approximately one third of men going through long-term chemotherapy. For this reason, your doctor will regularly look at your blood chemistry and other blood markers while you are being treated for cancer.

What are the signs and symptoms? As mentioned, an abnormally low white blood cell count, or more specifically neutrophil level, is fairly common while undergoing cancer treatment. A low neutrophil count can happen rapidly and can correct itself rapidly with medical assistance or time away from treatment.

However, when a low neutrophil count is accompanied by a fever (usually more than 100 degrees F° or 38 degrees C°), the situation is known as febrile neutropenia. This is a far more serious situation. The definition of febrile neutropenia is a fever of unknown origin without clinical or a documented source of infection (such as a bacteria or virus). Patients with this condition are at risk of a very serious infection that could require hospitalization or that can be life-threatening in rarer cases.

Patients that have a higher risk of fever and other signs of disease with neutropenia include:

- Patients 65 years or older (who generally have more immune issues)
- Patients with a poor performance status (see chapter one)
- Patients suffering from poor nutrition
- Those having an open wound or infection
- Patients who received extensive previous drug treatment
- Those receiving multiple or combination chemotherapies
- Those with a previous diagnosis of fever with neutropenia
- Patients with more advanced cancer
- Those having other disease (comorbidities) along with cancer

Other symptoms that can occur with neutropenia include chills, diarrhea or abdominal pain, dizziness, weakness, a general unwell feeling, or even severe cough. However, in many circumstances, a fever is the only sign of infections. Notify your doctor immediately if you develop a fever while on drug treatment for cancer, especially chemotherapy. Severe febrile neutropenia can delay cancer treatments or cause a dose reduction until it is brought under control.

Other more specific common sites of infection and symptoms include:

- Bladder—painful urination
- Gastrointestinal area—diarrhea, cramping, discomfort
- Lungs—cough, congestion, fluid coughed up that is yellow or green
- Nasal area—sinus pain, congestion, headache

- Rectal area—bleeding, pain when going to the bathroom
- Skin—redness, pain, tender or swelling near a cut or scratch

Prevention and Treatment Options

Lifestyle and Diet Tips

- Using an accurate thermometer, check your temperature any time that you do not feel well or are unusually warm. It is important to check your temperature while undergoing advanced cancer treatment, because often a temperature increase is the first sign of febrile neutropenia.
- Always wash your hands thoroughly with soap and water to prevent infections. Purchase a 62% ethyl alcohol hand gel. Use it regularly at home and in your travels in order to prevent infection. The ideal procedure is to first wash your hands and then use hand gel to ensure adequate prevention.
- Avoid individuals with colds, flu, or other illness. Consider avoiding crowds, young children or others who are or may be ill, and any other likely sources of infection when your blood counts are low.
- Prevent cuts or scrapes by wearing gloves. Keep any cut or scrape well bandaged and covered.
- Cook food thoroughly to kill any bacteria that may be on the raw food.
- Eat a generally healthy diet because it can help to maintain good immune health.
- Do not ingest products that advertise that they contain live microorganisms, such as some commercial kombucha teas.
- Especially in the fall and winter, use moisturizer or lotion from head to toe to prevent cracks in your skin or dry patches that can become irritated or infected. Chemotherapy and many other cancer treatments can dry the skin out, so it is smart to moisturize as much as possible to reduce itching and redness.

Dietary Supplements and Over-the-Counter Options

- Vitamin C dietary supplements have been studied to learn whether they improve the function of white blood cells because the concentration of vitamin C in them is many times higher as compared to most other cells of the human body. However, there is very little research on increased intake of vitamin C from supplements and its association with the risk of immune problems.

Prescriptions and Medical Procedures

- Regular monitoring of white blood cell counts by your doctor is recommended.
- Many chemotherapy drugs, but especially Taxotere, should not be administered unless the neutrophil blood count is over a certain number of cells as determined by your doctor. Some patients may be given broad spectrum antibiotics and use more precautions to prevent infection when their neutrophil counts go below a certain level.
- White blood cell–boosting drugs can be given at the beginning of, during, or even after chemotherapy if there is a problem with your white blood cell counts. One example of such a drug, G-CSF or GM-CSF (granulocyte macrophage-colony stimulating factor, also known as Sargramostim or Leukine) can be given as an injection to reduce the risk of blood disorders during treatment (including neutropenia or even febrile neutropenia). It is usually given by doctors who are concerned that patients might experience febrile neutropenia because they are at moderate to high risk of getting this condition.
- Other white blood cell count boosters include filgrastim (Neupogen) and pegfilgrastim (Neulasta). Filgrastim has to be taken more often than other medications such as pegfilgrastim. Talk to your doctor about which injection is needed for your situation (if any).
- The most common side effect that can occur from using these immune boosters is mild to moderate bone pain, which is usually controlled with a non-narcotic pain reliever such as acetaminophen (Tylenol). (Remember the Provenge immune-boosting treatment? Acetaminophen was given to every patient in the clinical trials before they received the therapy for this very reason.)
- Allergic-type reactions can occur with any white blood cell–boosting drug, such as rash, wheezing, drop in blood pressure,

swelling, pulse increase, and sweating. However, it is rare for this to happen (see the allergic reactions section).

NOSEBLEEDS

Also known as epistaxis.

What is it? Why does it happen? In cancer treatment, patients can have nosebleeds due to a low platelet count (known as thrombocytopenia). The body manufactures platelets to help with clotting or stop bleeding. Some cancer treatments and/or the cancer itself may increase the chance of problems with the platelets. A severely dry nose (mucosal dryness) can irritate blood vessels in the nose and cause bleeding in any individual. Medications that are placed in the nose can also irritate and dry the inside of the nose itself. Most common culprits are antihistamines or corticosteroids that are used for allergies or nasal congestion. Any blood-thinning drugs, such as warfarin, heparin, clopidogrel, and any non-steroidal anti-inflammatory drugs (NSAIDs) including aspirin and other over-the-counter pain relievers (not acetaminophen), can also cause nosebleeds. Trauma or an injury to the nose can be an issue, and dietary supplements, such as garlic and ginkgo biloba, can also cause the blood to thin and nose bleeds to occur.

Prevention and Treatment Options

Lifestyle and Diet Tips

- Talk to your doctor about blood-thinning drugs if you are having problems with nosebleeds.
- Using a humidifier in winter months when the air is dry may provide some relief.
- If you use nasal sprays, directing them laterally in each nostril away from the middle part of the nose can help reduce the risk of nosebleeds.
- Saline nasal sprays, used intermittently when the nose is dry may help. Some patients use a little petroleum jelly just inside each nostril to help keep the inside of the nose moist and reduce irritation and congestion.
- Avoid alcohol use because it can impact platelet function

and increase the risk for bleeding.

- If you are experiencing a nosebleed, you should sit upright, leaning slightly forward. Breathe through your mouth and apply direct pressure, pinching the outside portion of both nostrils closed using your thumb and index finger. Maintain pressure for at least 15 minutes. (Direct pressure along the nasal bones does not compress the blood vessels of the nose and stop bleeding.) Avoid tilting the head backwards because this can allow some blood to be swallowed or go down into the lungs. Once the bleeding stops, do not blow or disturb your nose. Avoid bending down for several hours as this might restart bleeding.

Dietary Supplements and Over-the-Counter Options

- In some cases, over-the-counter sinus congestion sprays containing oxymetazoline can help reduce the bleeding, particularly if the area begins to re-bleed a few hours later.

Prescriptions and Medical Procedures

If the bleeding does not stop easily or is concerning, patients should seek emergency care. There are many ways that health care professionals can stop nosebleeds using medication, cauterization, and nasal packing with materials that expand in the nostrils to cut off bleeding. It is always wise for cancer patients to discuss even mild nosebleeds with their health-care professionals to determine the best treatment for their individual situation.

PAIN

What is it? Why does it happen? Pain can be caused by cancer itself or it can be a side effect of cancer treatment. In the case of HRPC, tumors that have grown large enough to press on bone, surrounding tissues, organs, or nerves cause pain. It is also possible for cancer cells themselves to produce chemicals that may cause pain. Cancer treatments can also be responsible for some pain. For example, some chemotherapy treatments can cause tingling or numbness in the legs, arms, hands, or feet. On the other hand, an effective cancer treatment can also reduce pain by shrinking the cancer and taking pressure off a bone or nerve.

What are the signs and symptoms? We all know what it means to have pain, but it is important to give your doctor an accurate assessment of your pain. Commonly, a 1-to-10 scale is used, with 1 representing little or no pain and 10 being the worst possible pain you have ever experienced. Another way of considering it is that a score of 1 to 3 is mild pain, a score of 4 to 6 is moderate pain, and a score of 7 to 10 is severe pain. Mild pain can be treated usually with over-the-counter pain medications; moderate pain usually requires a prescription pain pill; and severe pain usually requires higher doses of prescription medications or perhaps an IV drug.

To begin, it is worth considering some common misconceptions about pain and prostate cancer.

Myth 1 HRPC means you will be in pain most of the time.

Fact 1 Only a small percentage of men with HRPC experience severe pain, and even then, often the pain is not there on a regular basis.

Myth 2 The doctor does not need to hear about every little ache or pain.

Fact 2 To provide you with the best care, the doctor does want and need to hear about any pain you experience. Your pain may be a symptom of a problem that needs to be treated, or it may be a symptom that qualifies you for another cancer treatment drug (not just a pain medication). Also, regardless of the intensity, pain saps energy and can alter your mood. No one benefits from avoiding discussion of the issue of pain with your doctor.

Myth 3 If you take pain medication or a regular basis, you will become addicted to or dependent on these drugs.

Fact 3 This is not the case. In many cases, the very strong pain medications are needed only for short intervals of time. When the medications are stopped, the majority of patients do not have a problem. In fact, one message from research that doctors are being taught right now is that the use of higher amounts of pain medication in cancer patients does not generally result in dependency or addiction for patients. In fact, it can improve both an individual's mental and physical health.

Myth 4 Only pain medications can reduce pain.

Fact 4 Not true. In reality, treating the underlying cause of the pain is very effective at reducing pain. When patients with pain experience a benefit from a cancer treatment, it is not unusual to experience a reduction in pain. For example, in the clinical trials with Taxotere chemotherapy, many men with pain who received a clinical benefit from the drug (tumor cells eliminated or tumors reduced in size) also felt a reduction in pain as the benefit occurred. Some were able to reduce their pain medications or come off of some pain medication completely. Therefore, it is important to realize that some cancer treatments not only can kill cancer cells but can also help reduce pain.

Myth 5 Pain medication is most effective when received intravenously.

Fact 5 Not necessarily. Pain medication should fit your personal situation. Some prefer to take pain pills, others like a lozenge or stick (like a lollipop), and others prefer a patch or another route that does not require taking pills. The truth is that when you are in control over the form or delivery system of the pain medication, it seems to improve mood and mental and physical health. You should not only tell your doctor when you think you need pain medication, but also request the type and form of pain medication that fits your personality and lifestyle.

Prevention and Treatment Options

Lifestyle and Diet Tips

- Exercise releases a natural painkiller endorphin that acts somewhat like an effective pain-reducing drug, but in a low concentration. Therefore, staying aerobically active (walking, jogging, swimming, rowing, or biking) is important in order to stay mentally and physically strong, and it may also work as a pain reliever by releasing endorphins.
- Resistance exercise or weightlifting should not be attempted without your doctor's approval because, in patients with bone metastasis, for example, it could increase the risk of pain and could cause a fracture.

Dietary Supplements and Over-the-Counter Options

- Mild pain can usually be controlled with over-the-counter pain medications, such as acetaminophen (Tylenol and generic) or a nonsteroidal anti-inflammatory drug (NSAID) such as ibuprofen (Advil, Motrin, etc.) or naproxen (Aleve). Keep in mind that acetaminophen can cause liver problems when combined with alcohol and that NSAIDs can make kidney problems or high blood pressure worse in some individuals. Also, these pills can upset the stomach, so make sure you take any over-the-counter pain pills with food.
- Acupuncture or acupressure—The strategic placement of needles or pressure at certain points of the body can cause the release of endorphins, the body's own pain-relieving chemicals. Some patients have found these treatments beneficial. However, they can also be expensive, so make sure you review price and consider how often you need treatment. Many of the clinical benefits are observed when just receiving treatment once every week or two. Additionally, many acupuncturists also sell herbal medicines, so you need to be careful about what you add to your current cancer treatment regimen.
- Aromatherapy—There are certain spas and clinics that specialize in aromatherapy, the science of using smells to cause a relaxing effect. This therapy may improve the patient's quality of life by reducing stress. It is an option for

some individuals who are looking for an alternative treatment to add to their conventional pain medication regimen.

- Biofeedback—Working with a technician in the area of biofeedback, an individual can control certain body functions, such as blood pressure, heart rate, and muscle tension. This can allow a person to relax and better deal with pain.
- Counseling and Support—Depression and anxiety can make a painful situation appear worse, so don't hesitate to ask for professional help. After a cancer diagnosis, individuals are given referrals to many professionals who can offer treatment, but often are not given the name of someone who can improve your mental health as you deal with the challenges of undergoing advanced cancer treatment.
- Guided Imagery—With this therapy, an individual uses his imagination to create mental pictures of more pleasant or less painful situations. Some people call guided imagery "deliberate daydreams." The underlying concept is to utilize the power of a patient's imagination to mentally change his circumstance and thereby lead to physical changes in his quality of life. Guided imagery can reduce stress, which in turn can reduce anxiety and improve mental health and energy.
- Applying heat and/or ice to a painful area may produce relief.
- Hypnosis—Some patients have experimented with hypnosis to manage pain.
- Massage—Some massage therapists specialize in chronic pain. You may want to try it if you have muscle soreness or discomfort that can be helped with massage therapy. Many patients feel massage has an added benefit of reducing stress.
- Some patients have had success with meditation or other relaxing alternative therapies (such as yoga).
- Creams, lotions, and gels that contain menthol can be soothing for pain in various parts of the body. However, read labels carefully as many of these products now contain aspirin or aspirin-like compounds as well. Those compounds can be absorbed into the blood in large amounts and result in undesirable blood thinning. Check with your

doctor to determine whether a menthol product with aspirin is okay or whether you should just stick with the menthol-only product.

- As we discussed in the neuropathy section, capsaicin cream or patch (with the active ingredient in hot chili peppers) can reduce neuropathic pain, so some patients may want to use it for pain that is near the surface of the skin. However, be careful and apply the product using gloves or a cotton swab. If you get capsaicin on your fingers and into your eyes, the burning sensation can be quite painful and potentially harmful.

Prescriptions and Medical Procedures

Pain Medication Delivery Systems

Prescription pain relievers come in a variety of forms to consider with your doctor:

- Intravenous injection (IV)
- Liquids
- Lollipop or stick
- Lozenges
- Nasal sprays
- Ointment (topical)
- Pump (controls delivery of medication)
- Patch (topical)
- Pills
- Suppository (rectal)

Pain Medication Frequency Options

Pain medications can be formulated to act over short and long periods of time. This is one reason why one medication may have several delivery options. Also, the variety of delivery options may be needed as an individual develops tolerance to the lower doses and requires a higher dose to provide a similar effect. Pain medication is sometimes dispensed on an "as needed" basis, which means that you take it when you think you need it. Immediate or rapid-acting pain medications exist if other options take too long to work. Long-lasting or extended-release forms of certain medications exist (morphine and oxycodone, for example). Skin patches that provide a steady dosage of pain medication (fentanyl) to the body all day long are also available.

Moderate pain can be controlled in some cases with higher doses of over-the-counter medications. However, if this is not working, your doctor may prescribe an opioid (narcotic) drug. Some of the more frequently used opioids include:

- Acetaminophen with codeine (Tylenol #2, #3, #4)
- Hydrocodone (Vicodin)
- Oxycodone (OxyContin or Percocet)
- Dihydrocodeine
- Propoxyphene
- NSAIDs with codeine, hydrocodone, or oxycodone
- Tramadol

Severe pain can be treated with a stronger opioid drug (keep in mind that the doctor may also recommend an over-the-counter pain reliever or another drug with these medications). Some options used are:

- Fentanyl (the Duragesic patch, for example) and other closely related medications
- Hydromorphone (Dilaudid)
- Levorphanol (similar to morphine)
- Methadone
- Morphine (Contin)
- Oxycodone (OxyContin)

Other pain treatment options involve the use of radiation. Radiopharmaceuticals (such as Samarium-153 [Quadramet] and Strontium-89 [Metastron]) are administered in an IV. They locate the tumor and deliver radiation to it. Also, spot radiation can be delivered only to the site of a tumor, for example on a bone, and can reduce PSA and pain.

Pain Medication Side Effects

- Constipation can be a common side effect of pain medication. Increasing fluid and fiber intake can help prevent this from happening, or your doctor may suggest or prescribe a laxative drug.
- Nausea and vomiting or stomach upset can occur. Taking pain medications with food and using ground ginger (1/4 to

1/2 teaspoon a day) or 500 to 1000 mg of ginger dietary supplements can help reduce the frequency of this side effect.

- Drowsiness is another issue with some pain medications. Having a caffeinated beverage with or around the time you take your pain medication may alleviate this problem.
- Generally speaking, reducing or dividing the dosage of pain medication is always a possibility if any of the side effects of pain medication are a real problem.Talk to your doctor about this possibility.

PENIS AND SCROTUM SHRINKAGE

Also known as genital atrophy.

What is it? Why does it happen? There are nerve bundles that run along the prostate and help to control erections. If any of them are injured or become less active, there is less of a connection to the penis and scrotum, and thus less stimulus. This can result in a small change in length and/or width of the penis. Additionally, male hormone helps maintain the size of the genital area, so when testosterone is reduced this can also potentially reduce the size of the penis and scrotum area. Any treatment that may affect the nerves near the prostate and/or male hormone levels could potentially slightly affect penis size. Therefore, most prostate cancer treatments, from surgery to radiation to ADT, could potentially have this impact. Talk to your doctor about it and how it can be prevented.

Prevention and Treatment Options

Prescriptions and Medical Procedures

The "use it or lose it" characteristic of the human body can help prevent this problem. This means talking to your doctor about regularly using any of the erectile dysfunction treatment methods discussed earlier in this chapter in order to continue to maintain nerve stimulation and the length and width of the penis. Men have used pills, injections, pumps, and other methods not only to improve erectile function but to make sure that there is no reduction in size of the genital area. If the nerves have to be eliminated because of the cancer, talk to your doctor about what you can do about this condition.

STRESS AND ANXIETY

Note In some cases, stress and anxiety can also be associated with depression (see the depression section). If there is a concern that any of these conditions (stress, anxiety, or depression) may be seriously affecting you, then you should seek treatment from a professional. Stress, anxiety, and depression are all medically distinct conditions. However, stress and anxiety often overlap, so they have been grouped together in this section.

What is it? Why does it happen? Stress and anxiety can range in severity from the average day-to-day issues of dealing with cancer to feelings that can reach a level that affects physical and mental health, and your quality of life. For some reason, mental health improvement has always taken a real back seat to physical health improvement during cancer treatment. However, it is important to recognize the tie between physical and mental health. Finances, cancer, job, family, fitness level, and virtually every other aspect of your life can affect how you feel or deal with life physically.

What are the signs and symptoms? The body responds to stress by releasing greater amounts of many hormones and compounds that can be bad for your health in general. For example, the adrenal glands release excessive amounts of norepinephrine, epinephrine, and cortisol when there is chronic stress. While having some of these hormones is normally helpful, they are unhealthy in excess. Stress can cause your heart rate, blood pressure, and blood sugar levels to increase, which can increase the risk of cardiovascular problems. Stress can also reduce the strength of your immune system by causing a reduction in specific types of cells and antibodies that normally fight infections. Stress can cause muscular tension, nervousness, and headaches (especially tension headaches). It can impair your memory, disrupt focus and concentration, and make it difficult to get adequate sleep or rest, which means it can cause both mental and physical fatigue. Recently, research has even demonstrated that stress can reduce the quantity of healthy bacteria found in your gastrointestinal tract and cause digestive problems. From head to toe, chronic stress can have a negative impact on your life.

Prevention and Treatment Options

Lifestyle and Diet Tips

- Never be shy about seeking medical attention or therapy from a professional (social worker, therapist, psychiatrist, regular physician, other health care worker, religious counselor, etc.) for your stress, because treating stress can have a dramatic and immediate impact on improving your life. Cognitive Behavioral Therapy (CBT) has been found to work as well as some medications when used appropriately in working with a medical professional. CBT involves regular advice and suggestions that allow a person to move away from feeling regular stress or anxiety.
- There are numerous stress questionnaires available on the Internet that can be printed and filled out and given to your health care professional so that your stress can be somewhat quantified. For example, the Perceived Stress Scale (PSS) tries to determine how much stress has impacted your life over the last month. Answering these questions not only helps you to understand how you are doing, but is also empowering and therapeutic because understanding this issue helps you to start taking control of your situation.
- There are also other ways to evaluate your stress. Consider some of the following basic questions (and please share with your health care professional):
  - How would you describe your energy level?
  - How have you been sleeping?
  - How has your mood been lately?
  - What kind of pressure have you been dealing with at work, home, or in general?
  - What do you do to unwind at the end of the day, and do you have difficulty unwinding?
  - To whom do you turn for support?

- Are there any personal issues that need to be covered that you would like to share with your health care professional?
- Keep a diary or notebook by your bed to write down things that are generating stress for you. These can be shared with your health care professional.
- Consider bringing a companion to your medical visits, because this person can help you to remember things at the visit, including questions you may have and the doctor's recommendations. This can reduce stress. (Some individuals even bring a tape recorder.) A companion or close friend reduces stress because discussing concerns is therapeutic.
- Get an organizer or binder to keep all your medical information in one organized place. This will help you to gain some control, become more empowered, and feel less stressed.
- Allow yourself to experiment with other not-so-heavily-advertised stress-reducing activities. Consider if one of the following might suit you: joining a support group, journaling, art therapy, guided imagery, hypnosis, music therapy, horticultural therapy, meditation, tai chi, or yoga. Many of these opportunities are offered free of charge at centers such as the Wellness Community, Gilda's House, etc. They not only provide you with support but can assist your family as well. Pick the one that might fit your personality best, and give it a try. It is interesting that one of the top selling over-the-counter devices to reduce blood pressure teaches you how to lower blood pressure by slowing your breathing and relaxing (controlled respiration). The stress-reducing activities above can work by allowing you to gain control over your situation and physiology, and the body actually responds by reducing blood pressure, heart rate, and stress!
- Any diet or activity that reduces blood pressure can also reduce anxiety, which is another reason eating a low-sodium and healthy diet may actually be a benefit.
- Alcohol and tobacco are often used to relax or temporarily reduce stress. In reality, once the anti-stress effect goes away,

the body responds by significantly increasing the quantity of stress hormones that it produces. Also, over time, the body develops resistance to these compounds so that higher doses are needed to relax you. A roller coaster of dependency is created. So, keep your alcohol intake to moderate levels and eliminate tobacco products.

- Similarly, high consumption of caffeine can also cause a dependency that only increases stress with greater use. Certain unhealthy foods can have the same effect by making you feel good in the short term but increasing stress in the long term.
- Medications (supplement and prescriptions) can cause you to completely rely on a pill for a temporary solution. For that reason, a pill should be used only when lifestyle changes and therapy are not effective by themselves.
- Fitness or exercise is one of the best ways to reduce stress and anxiety. The body responds to exercise by reducing your heart rate, blood pressure, and blood sugar. It also releases endorphins, which are compounds associated with a state of relaxation and improved mood. You've heard of a "runner's high"? That is really an anti-stress exercise phenomenon.

Dietary Supplements and Over-the-Counter Options

Note *Any anti-stress supplement combined with medications already given by your doctor to reduce stress, anxiety, or depression may cause a drug interaction that can be dangerous. Always check with your doctor or pharmacist to make sure there are no potential negative drug interactions. Also, sudden withdrawal of a supplement or drug that can reduce stress and blood pressure may create danger by causing a dramatic increase in blood pressure or heart rate, so a gradual withdrawal always makes more sense.*

- L-theanine is the best anti-stress supplement option when used at a dose of 200 to 250 mg per day. It is backed by many preliminary studies that show it is safe and effective at this dosage. Some supplement companies are combining this ingredient with numerous other ingredients in order to have a unique blend, but this ignores the fact that L-theanine by itself was used in the most effective clinical trials. The other interesting feature of L-theanine is that it comes from green tea. It is believed that L-theanine helps to counteract the stimulatory effects of caffeine in tea. L-theanine has a great safety record and has been used as an additive in candy, foods, and beverages in Japan for decades. Doses even as low as 50 mg of L-theanine in some beverages have provided anti-stress relief.

- GABA (gamma-amino butyric acid) is a compound that works in the brain to reduce stress and anxiety. It is now sold as an effective dietary supplement that will probably be found to work as well as any other dietary supplement for stress, simply based on the fact that this compound has been used for a long time in other countries. Doses of only 50 to 200 mg per day of this supplement have been effective in preliminary studies. Side effects of this medication have not been determined because most studies have not followed individuals over the long term. But remember that any anti-stress product carries at least the potential for drug interaction and dependency.
- Bacopa monniera (also known as Brahmi or just Bacopa) is an alternative Ayurvedic medicine. In preliminary clinical trials of doses of 300 mg per day, it reduced stress and anxiety better than a placebo. This supplement comes in a liquid or syrup form and may also have blood pressure–lowering effects. This is not surprising; any time a product reduces stress, many of the physiologic measurements associated with stress improve with it (blood pressure and heart rate, for example).
- Other stress supplements such as Rhodiola rosea (SHR-5) at 50 mg twice a day, fish oil, and even L-tyrosine have all been promoted to reduce stress, but they need more research.
- Valerian is not a good anti-stress or anti-anxiety supplement; it is a sleep aid, and it has drug interactions. Taking a sleeping pill to reduce stress is not usually advisable.

Prescriptions and Medical Procedures

- Cognitive behavioral therapy (CBT) or working with a medical professional in combination with medication is arguably the most effective combination. In some cases where the combination is used, no medication is needed at all. In fact, regular behavioral intervention or recommendations from a therapist can have a positive impact that is as good as any supplement or drug.
- That being said, there are several drugs and drug classes that are very effective for anxiety and stress, including benzodiazepine medications such as alprazolam (Xanax), clonazepam (Klonopin), diazepam (Valium), lorazepam (Ativan), and oxazepam (Serax). They reduce nerve activity in the brain and can work quickly to provide a calming effect, but they can also make you sleepy and should not be combined with alcohol.
- Buspirone (Buspar) is a drug that is generally not addictive and does not make you sleepy, but it can take longer to work.
- In some cases, antidepressants are also effective for anxiety and stress, especially when these problems are also accompanied by some depression.
- Blood pressure and heart rate-lowering medications (such as beta-blockers) may also be recommended in some cases for anxiety. There is a long list of medications, and your doctor can advise you as to which might be best for your situation.

SWEATING

Also known as hyperhidrosis.

What is it? Why does it happen? Sweating an abnormal amount at unpredictable times is not always the result of an extreme temperature change, but it may be a side effect of some cancer treatments or other medications. The condition usually impacts the palms of the hands, soles of the feet and/or underarms.

Prevention and Treatment Options

Lifestyle and Diet Tips

- Loose-fitting natural fiber clothing, such as cotton, wool, and silk, can allow your skin to breathe and feel cooler.

- Be careful not to use moisturizer on areas prone to sweating as it can make the condition worse.
- Relaxation techniques, such as paced, controlled respiration, yoga, or meditation, can help since stress can make the problem worse.
- Review the section on hot flashes as episodes of sweating may be due to hot flashes. Remedies suggested there to reduce hot flashes will also improve sweating if it is actually due to hot flashes.

Dietary Supplements and Over-the-Counter Options

- Often, applying antiperspirant to the affected areas will improve the condition.

Prescriptions and Medical Procedures

Health care professionals have many options for hyperhidrosis that cannot be controlled simply by over-the-counter options.

- Prescription antiperspirants that are made of concentrated (10-15%) aluminum chloride can be applied at night on the area of concern and washed off in the morning to prevent excessive drying and irritation of the area. A benefit may be realized with only short-term use of these antiperspirants.
- A hydrocortisone cream is sometimes used on these areas during the day.
- There are also several anticholinergic drugs that doctors can prescribe to cause a general drying effect. However, they do have other side effects when taken as a pill (drowsiness, constipation, urinary retention) so this is not the best way to get them. When added to tap water, anticholinergics can be applied directly to the sweat glands of the problem area, reducing the chance for unintended side effects.
- Iontophoresis, a low-energy electrical current applied to the specific sweating area (usually by a dermatologist), can also work. However, it is time consuming and it does have potential side effects (skin irritation, pain, blistering). Patients may have difficulty locating a doctor who has the device.
- In rare cases, Botox injections, different forms of surgery, or out-patient procedures are also effective.

TASTE CHANGES

Also known as dysgeusia.

What is it? Why does it happen? This is an abnormal taste, an unpleasant change in the sense of taste, or even an alteration in a taste sensation. This is a generally unrecognized side effect of Taxotere and some other chemotherapy medications including:

- Carboplatin
- Cisplatin
- Cyclophosphamide
- Dacarbazine
- Dactinomycin
- Doxorubicin
- 5-flurouracil
- Levamisole
- Mechlorethamine
- Paclitaxel
- Vincristine

Taste changes may be caused by temporary nerve damage from the cancer drug itself that may also affect taste receptors. Another possibility is that receptor cells can be damaged so that there is a decrease in the number of receptor cells, or a change in the cell receptor may occur. Human taste bud cells are replenished every 10 days, and the smell receptor cells life span is only about a week. With radiation to some areas of the body and some chemotherapy agents destroying cells that replicate quickly, it makes sense that there may be an influence on taste bud or smell receptor cells in some patients. In addition, certain cancer drugs themselves contain bitter-tasting compounds. Other possible factors causing taste changes can include infections, postnasal drip, acid reflux, mouth sores (see the stomatitis section), and even improper oral hygiene. Depression and stress can also make the problem worse because these conditions are associated with a lack of interest in proper nutrition.

Dry mouth is also a common cause of taste changes

during cancer treatment. In addition to chemotherapy drugs, many other drugs can reduce the amount of saliva produced by the body. Talk to your doctor about other medications, such as antihistamines and anti-inflammatory drugs, that can contribute to drying.

What are the signs and symptoms? Changes in taste can be described as a metallic, bitter, salty, or simply unpleasant. This problem is closely associated with changes in smell, because taste and smell are both involved in giving someone a sensation of taste. This problem can affect quality of life by increasing the risk of poor nutrition and weight loss. In the clinic or laboratory, it can be officially evaluated by a health care professional. She or he will determine any impact on the five basic human tastes—sweetness, bitterness, sourness, saltiness, and the savoriness of protein-rich foods (also known as umami). A simpler diagnosis is based solely on patient reports of symptoms. This problem can last for days, weeks, or even longer depending on the frequency of chemotherapy.

Prevention and Treatment Options

Lifestyle and Diet Tips

- Nutritional counseling has been moderately effective in several randomized studies, so please talk to your qualified cancer nutritionist about some suggestions. A consultation with a qualified dietician can also make suggestions on how to overcome specific taste changes, still eat well, and maintain proper nutrition.
- Cooking decisions, such as marinating meat or using soy sauces, juices, certain salad dressings, table wine, or other items, may help to mask any abnormal smell or taste. Flavor food when possible with spices, herbs, sugar, and sauces.
- Chewing gums, mints, or even lemon drop candy may increase saliva production in the mouth before eating, which can improve the sensation of taste.
- If taste changes are more severe, an individual can consume foods with a milder flavor that are nutritious and high in protein, such as fish, chicken, dairy products, and egg whites.

- If food has a metallic taste, switching to plastic utensils may help.
- Nutritional liquid supplements can substitute for some meals. On average, they should contain 20 grams of protein and 200 calories per serving, so look for these at your local pharmacy or health food store.
- There have been a few reports of using ice cube stimulation to improve taste changes. Individuals were told to leave a small amount of crushed ice or ice cubes in the mouth and on their tongue for 1 minute before every meal, and this has helped some regain normal taste. This method was also discussed as a useful option to prevent mouth sores (see the mouth sores section). It seems that taste receptors may not only be sensitive to taste, but also to temperature. When the temperature of the mouth increases after removal of the ice, it is possible that blood circulation increases to this area, helping in some way to improve taste.
- Dry mouth may increase the risk of taste changes, and it may simply make things worse by itself. Saliva not only improves taste and digestion, but also provides an immune healthy benefit and prevents infections of all types, including those caused by bacteria and especially yeast/fungus. Keeping the mouth moist with saliva substitutes or stimulants that can be purchased over the counter is a good idea if you have dry mouth. These substitutes and stimulants come in sprays, liquids, lozenges, and even gels. They are loaded with many of the same or similar ingredients found in natural saliva, but they carry none of the digestive benefits. Keep in mind that tobacco, too much alcohol, or caffeine can make things worse because these are diuretics that can increase dry mouth. Also, please keep in mind that acupuncture is backed by some preliminary evidence that it can treat dry mouth.

Dietary Supplements and Over-the-Counter Options

While there is no standard or accepted preventative or simple treatment for taste changes, some of the same reasons taste changes occur is due to the same type of nerve damage that causes peripheral neuropathy. It may be that by treating or preventing peripheral neuropathy with alpha-lipoic acid or another medication, taste changes can be minimized.

In a non-cancer study of zinc gluconate (140 mg per day) for individuals with taste changes, the supplement did show some benefit and also a surprise improvement in mood as compared to a placebo. However, in a recently published study, zinc sulfate (45 mg 3 times a day for a total of 135 mg) supplements did not work significantly better than a placebo in cancer patients receiving radiation therapy who experienced taste changes, but there were some minor-to-modest overall benefits in the zinc group that were almost statistically significant. Zinc gluconate pills or lozenges have a better safety record than zinc sulfate, so zinc gluconate may be worth a try. However, 140 mg per day is a very large dosage. If you experience taste changes, consider (with your doctor) starting low doses of 30 mg per day and increasing the dose by another 20 to 30 mg every week. If the problem gets better or goes away, it would make sense to stop supplementing with high doses of zinc because really high doses of zinc can cause gastrointestinal problems. Most health care professionals also recommend at least 1 to 2 mg of copper supplementation with higher zinc intakes taken for longer periods of time (months) to prevent a rare form of anemia. Most children's multivitamins contain this amount of copper. Many zinc supplements also contain copper. Never use zinc nasal sprays, gels, or any product that has you put zinc into the nose because these products can cause you to permanently lose sense of smell and taste.

A recent study testing doses of 30 grams of the popular dietary supplement glutamine did not improve taste changes.

Prescriptions and Medical Procedures

There are no safe and effective medications for taste loss from cancer treatment, but there are a few options for dry mouth.

- Pilocarpine stimulates saliva flow, but it also causes a number of other changes such as increases in sweating, tears, and urinary frequency.
- Another medication cevimeline (Evoxac), has so many

head-to-toe side effects that it should be used only for moderate to severe dry mouth that has no other solutions.

- Amifostine is a sulfur-based compound that protects normal organs and tissues from free radical or oxidative damage caused by some cancer therapies. However, this popular drug has not been effective in reducing taste changes, so it should not be used for this problem.

TESTOSTERONE DEFICIENCY SYNDROME

Also known as androgen deprivation syndrome or male menopause syndrome.

What is it? Why does it happen? This is a rare occurrence. In fact, it is so rare that there really is not an adequate name for it. Most men with HRPC have been carrying a castrate level of testosterone (virtually no testosterone) for some time. It is always hard to predict the impact of this "male menopause" on the overall quality of life of any man. In some cases, dramatic changes take place that simply cannot be addressed by any side-effect medication, except for getting some testosterone itself. Of course, it is rare to receive testosterone during prostate cancer treatment, but it does happen, and the question needs to be addressed.

What are the signs and symptoms? There are HRPC situations in which an individual needs some testosterone again for a short period of time because his testosterone deficiency syndrome is causing a multitude of problems (fatigue, weakness, discomfort, muscle loss). This is a quality-of-life decision that several prostate cancer experts recommend in rare situations. It is important to know that the longer a man is on ADT, the less likely it is that he will ever naturally produce testosterone again. The only way for these men to get testosterone is through an outside medication. Of course, there are catches with using testosterone, such as a potential cardiac risk in a high-risk person, stimulation of tumor growth, and other issues that your doctor should discuss with you.

Prevention and Treatment Options

Lifestyle and Diet Tips

There are no lifestyle changes that can dramatically increase your testosterone. However, there are certain lifestyle changes, such as weight loss, associated with a greater chance of observing a slight testosterone increase.

Dietary Supplements and Over-the-Counter Options

There is one testosterone-making dietary supplement, DHEA, which is inadequate at making large enough amounts of testosterone unless a person is willing to take several hundred milligrams of it daily. It generally is not recommended for testosterone replacement therapy because it is not as efficient as receiving testosterone itself. And any time a person takes a hormone pill, especially DHEA or even a testosterone pill, it increases the chances of liver or cardiovascular problems. A final concern with DHEA pills, aside from the fact that they can stimulate tumor growth is that in some men DHEA is converted more into estrogen than into testosterone, so the desired effect is not achieved.

Prescriptions and Medical Procedures

There are multiple testosterone replacement therapy (TRT) options today, including:

- Testosterone gel (transdermal delivery of testosterone). This therapy requires daily application to clean, dry skin in the shoulder or stomach area. The gel is allowed to dry completely before dressing. Since the gel can be transferred to family members, it is recommended that you wash your hands thoroughly after using it.
- Testosterone injection into muscle. This tends to be lower in cost, but injections are needed about every 2 weeks. While it is easy to achieve the maximum level of testosterone in the blood, a "roller coaster" effect can also occur between injections. There is a variety of dosages available. Pain at the injection site is possible.
- Testosterone patch (transdermal delivery of testosterone). Scrotal and non-scrotal skin patches are available, and daily

application is needed (The patch delivers 5 to 10 mg per day). Skin irritation or inadequate absorption through the skin can be a problem for some individuals.
- Testosterone pellets (inserted by a physician in his office). Testospel in 75 mg doses is one currently available product. Several pellets are placed just under the skin in the hip area or the upper buttocks just below the beltline. The procedure takes about 10 minutes, and no stitches are needed, but the doctor does have to numb the area with a local anesthetic. Delivers testosterone for 3 to 6 months.
- Buccal testosterone (Striant) A tablet-shaped patch applied to the upper gum area. Talk to your doctor.
- Testosterone pills (oral). These are not usually prescribed because this type of testosterone comes with an increased risk of causing liver problems (hepatotoxicity). Although they are offered over the Internet, they are not safe and should be avoided.

THROMBOCYTOPENIA

Also known as low platelet count

What is it? Why does it happen? Thrombocytes (also know as platelets) are fragments of bone marrow cells found in the blood. They play a crucial role in stopping bleeding, both on the surface and inside the body. A low platelet count is usually a side effect of chemotherapy. As has been previously discussed, chemotherapy can be toxic to rapidly dividing cells, both cancerous and normal body cells Bone marrow is one of the normal cells that may be affected negatively by chemotherapy and a drop in the number of platelets may occur as a result.

Prevention and Treatment Options

Lifestyle and Diet Tips

- Avoid situations where injury might occur if possible. Bleeding or bruising may be difficult to stop so avoiding situations prone to causing injury are preferred. You

should do only low-impact exercises such as walking or swimming if a doctor determines your platelet count is low.
- Shaving with an electric razor may eliminate the chance of a cut.
- Use a soft-bristle toothbrush to avoid damage to the inside of the mouth.
- Avoid alcohol use as it can reduce platelet counts even further.

Prescriptions and Medical Procedures

- Physicians may recommend slowing treatment schedules to allow platelet counts to naturally increase again.
- More severe cases may be treated using a platelet transfusion from a blood bank. There is a risk of an allergic reaction from receiving platelets as a transfusion but the benefit is greater than the risk here if your doctor determines that the additional platelets are needed.

TINGLING AND NUMBNESS

Also known as paresthesia and citrate toxicity.

What is it? Why does it happen? Paresthesia is the sensation of tingling, prickling, or numbness of the skin, often around the mouth. The feeling is often similar to the feeling one gets when a part of the body falls asleep. There are many causes of paresthesia, but it is fairly common in HRPC patients undergoing leukapheresis (see chapter five on Provenge treatment). During the process, a citrate compound is used to prevent components of the blood from sticking together as a patient's immune cells are harvested. However, citrate can lower the level of calcium in the blood temporarily and cause a hypersensitive nerve sensation known as a paresthesia. While it generally causes no long-term problems, paresthesia could make it difficult for patients to recover from a treatment or receive another treatment.

What is it? Why does it happen? Tingling, prickling, or numbness of the skin surrounding the mouth following a leukapherisis procedure.

Prevention and Treatment Options

Lifestyle and Diet Tips

Interestingly, several small studies have shown that giving calcium carbonate dietary supplements (1000 to 1500 mg per day) soon after the leukaphresis procedure is completed may reduce the risk of this toxicity by supplying the blood with more calcium. This is good advice for men with HRPC receiving a leukaphresis procedure because bone loss is generally a concern. However, men who regularly take calcium citrate supplements for bone loss prevention could theoretically increase the risk of paresthesia or make it worse. Therefore, men receiving leukapheresis should avoid calcium citrate and instead take 1000 to 1200 mg of calcium carbonate supplements daily throughout the treatment process, including a week after it has been completed. Talk to your doctor about making this change to help reduce the risk of paresthesias after leukapheresis.

WATERY EYES

Also known as excessive tearing, epiphora, dacryostenosis, or canalicular stenosis.

What is it? Why does it happen? This is a less common side effect of Taxotere chemotherapy (only about 10 percent of patients experience it), but its occurrence increases the more frequently Taxotere is given to the patient. In general, excessive tearing is due to a narrowing or inflammation and potential blockage of the area of the eye that drains the tears (the eye duct). As a result, the natural lubrication or fluid covering and protecting the eye cannot drain, and it spills out on the face and cheeks.

Some cancer medications that can also cause tearing include:

- Arsenic trioxide
- Cytarabine
- **Docetaxel (Taxotere)**
- Doxorubicin
- Epirubicin
- Fluorouracil

- Ifosfamide
- Methotrexate
- Mitoxantrone
- Oxaliplatin
- Paclitaxel
- Pentostatin
- Thiotepa

What are the signs and symptoms? This problem is exactly as it sounds and simply results in abnormal production of tears or fluid from the eyes. The tearing can be mild and barely noticeable or, in some cases, cause someone to continuously wipe tears off the face and eyes. Keep in mind that most cases of tearing from chemotherapy tend to be mild, do not need treatment, and get better over time. However, when someone is concerned about the problem or does need treatment, there are multiple solutions.

Prevention and Treatment Options

Lifestyle and Diet Tips

- "Reflex tearing," or tearing that is caused by allergies, irritants, infections, or other eye problems, may only increase the patient's annoyance. Therefore, anything that can further irritate the eyes during this time, such as smoke, exhaust, pollution, dust, pollen, and contact lenses that are not adequately taken care of, should be avoided if possible.

Dietary Supplements and Over-the-Counter Options

- Ocular moisturizers, such as Artificial Tears (lubricant eye drops) and 0.9% sodium chloride (preservative free to avoid eye irritation) can reduce eye irritation. It may sound odd to add moisture to eyes to help correct excessive tearing, but reducing irritation can help reduce tear production. Artificial tears can be used throughout the day to moisturize and provide relief. Do remember to look for the words "preservative free" on the label. These products may be most helpful when used for general prevention and also around the time of Taxotere administration. In fact, a recent study of artificial tears as compared to eye steroids (see following) found that they were equally effective in most patients.

- Anti-inflammatory pain medication could theoretically reduce the inflammation that is occurring in the tear duct, but this has not been adequately tested.
- Omega-3 (fish oil) and omega-6 dietary supplements have been shown by research to help with eye lubrication and in preventing the eyes from becoming too dry. If you have excessive tearing from chemotherapy, you may want to consider cutting back or eliminating these supplements until the condition gets better. However, there is no research that demonstrates whether or not the excess eye fluid stimulated from omega fatty acid supplements is good or bad for the excessive tearing situation. Perhaps since fish oil supplements appear to reduce inflammation they could be a potential benefit if the tearing situation is mild. In the absence of research, you will need to decide with your doctor what is best for your situation.

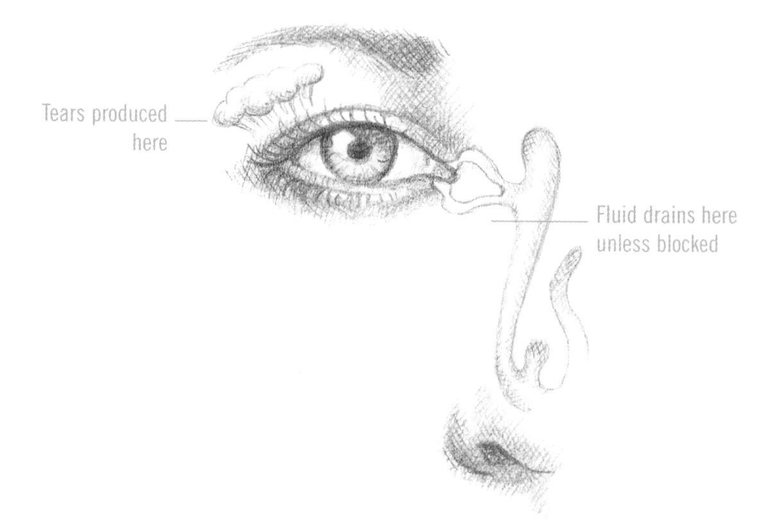

Prescriptions and Medical Procedures

- An eye specialist or ophthalmologist can be seen as needed before chemotherapy begins or if excessive tearing occurs.
- A simple "probing and irrigation" of the affected area can be done by the eye doctor with a tiny medical instrument. Sometimes this is all that is needed to resolve the problem.
- Topical eye steroids or a combination product that also has

an antimicrobial compound in it may be helpful when some symptoms arise. Eye steroid drops should be used carefully and for the shortest possible time because the drug itself could slightly increase the risk of other problems if used for very long periods of time (such as infections, nerve issues, and vision problems). Increasing the total steroid dosage with chemotherapy by adding an additional steroid is not generally a good idea because it may increase the risk of other problems in the rest of the body (infections, lower blood counts, etc.).

- Surgical insertion (a simple outpatient procedure) of silicone stents (silicone intubation) in the nasolacrimal duct nexts to the eyes to keep them open so they can drain the tears can be helpful in rare cases where this condition cannot be managed by medications. These tiny tubes are just inserted temporarily until the entire course of chemotherapy has concluded and they can be removed at anytime.
- Interesting experimental therapies available right now include Botox injection into each eye tear duct area (lacrimal gland). This makes some sense in rare cases because Botox has been used to weaken overactive muscles or to control excessive release of certain compounds, for example, excessive sweating. It has also helped some patients who have excessive tearing from causes other than chemotherapy by temporarily shutting off the production of a compound that causes tearing, with effects noticeable within about a week. However, these injections are not inexpensive, and other side effects, such as double vision and drooping of the eyelid, can occur. These injections are not commonly used for this condition.
- In rare and severe cases of complete or total narrowing of the eye ducts and excessive tearing that cannot be improved with any other intervention, there is another procedure known as conjunctivodacryocystorhinostomy. It is accomplished by inserting a tiny permanent Pyrex glass tube (also known as a Jones tube) into each duct

to overcome the blockage problem. This procedure is rarely needed, but helpful to those who need it.

WEIGHT GAIN

What is it? Why does it happen? Testosterone helps to drive metabolism. The hormone makes it easier to maintain or increase muscle mass and reduces the chances of excess weight gain. However, most men with HRPC have to remain on ADT or testosterone-suppressive treatment, so they tend to gain substantial amounts of weight and expand their waistlines unless aggressive preventive measures are utilized.

What are the signs and symptoms? Several measures of weight can increase during cancer treatment. Body mass index (BMI), total weight in general, the amount of fat in the body, and waist circumference (WC) or belly fat (especially fat under the skin, or subcutaneous fat) can all increase, frustrating men who experience it.

In this section, we will focus on weight loss strategies that are heart healthy as opposed to those that may have unhealthy side effects, such as increased heart rate or blood pressure, cholesterol increases, or feelings of stress or depression. Your overall health is of the first importance, particularly during cancer treatment.

Prevention and Treatment Options

Lifestyle and Diet Tips

- Consuming alcohol in moderate to high amounts results in many non-nutritional calories. Eliminating or cutting back on alcohol intake is often an easy way to lose weight if you are willing.
- Exercising daily, even at moderate levels, is a great way to burn calories as well as obtain a host of other health benefits. If your doctor gives you the okay, adding resistance exercise (such as weight lifting) to your routine 2 or 3 days a week increases your muscle mass, which will also increase your metabolism.
- Green tea and other teas have no calories, can be served

hot or cold, and are good to add to your weight loss program. Avoid sugary drinks that are loaded with calories.

- Reducing your total daily caloric intake by 250 to 500 calories per day allows most individuals to lose a pound every week or two, or at least to maintain their weight.
- Fiber, particularly insoluble fiber found in All-Bran, Fiber One, and other cereals, helps you feel full and provides other healthy benefits. A 1/3 cup serving of All-Bran with some flaxseed or chia seed added provides 15 to 20 grams of fiber—a great start toward your goal of 25 to 30 grams of fiber a day. Dietary fiber sources are better first choices than fiber pills. (See the constipation section for foods that are high in fiber.)

Dietary Supplements and Over-the-Counter Options

- Several studies suggest that fish oil dietary supplements taken in small amounts daily (with 1000 to 2000 mg a day of the active ingredients EPA and DHA) seem to promote weight loss and are heart healthy (they lower triglycerides). Keep in mind that fish oil can act as a blood thinner in some individuals, especially those taking other more potent blood thinners, so talk to your doctor.
- Combination "fat" appetite suppressant "shots" or small drinks now exist. For example, a combination of oat and palm oils (with monounsaturated and saturated fat) is commercially available. This may have some limited benefit, for a small concentration of fat (monounsaturated, polyunsaturated, and/or saturated fat) tends to send a signal to the brain that helps control appetite. However, other less expensive options might include taking a teaspoon or two of canola, olive, or safflower oil, or perhaps a spoonful of peanut butter. These options appear safe and may provide some small benefits in the short term.
- Dietary supplement protein powders can be mixed with low- or no-calorie liquids (including water) They include whey protein and egg white protein powder. They at least provide a health benefit by providing high-quality protein, making you feel more full, and potentially reducing muscle

loss. Whey protein comes in 3 basic forms—a concentrate (the cheapest), isolate, and hydrolysate/micronized (the most expensive). They are similar, except that the concentrate carries a greater chance of causing an allergy if you are allergic or sensitive to dairy products. The isolate, and especially the hydrolysate, are less allergenic for some individuals. Additionally, individuals who have some digestive problems should purchase the isolate or hydrolysate because this form of whey protein has already been partially broken up into smaller fragments, making it easier to absorb. If you want to go with a strictly vegetarian protein powder, there are also soy protein and brown rice protein powders now. They are also wonderful choices. Just a serving or two a day is nutritious, low in calorie, and may curb appetite.

- Some fiber supplements have Glucomannan (one of the most researched fibers) as an ingredient. This fiber can help with appetite suppression, weight loss, and some sugar control. However, cost is an issue. Also, these pills expand slightly in the stomach, which means they could also expand in your throat. Always take any fiber pills or product with a full glass of water.
- Modified citrus pectin (MCP) is another fiber powder option that contains a lot of fiber, but can be costly.
- "Resistant starch" can be purchased in bulk. It is actually another type of fiber that your body cannot absorb. It is found in foods such as navy beans, lentils, and cooked potatoes. It can be added to food and some beverages to give you that fiber-full feel (but why not just use fiber?).
- Orlistat (Alli) is an over-the-counter drug that is sold as a prescription in higher doses. It is a drug that blocks the absorption of dietary fat. The dose is one 60-milligram pill with meals three times a day. You also need to take a children's multivitamin daily because you will not be able to absorb certain important nutrients when there is less fat absorption. Orlistat can be expensive, but it may help you drop several pounds or more. Keep in mind that the fat in

the diet that you do not absorb goes right out the other end. To be fair, this side effect improves over time.

- Green tea supplements contain a popular compound known as EGCG. It is advertised as the calorie-burning compound in green tea that increases metabolism. However, many studies used 300 milligrams per day in capsules along with higher amounts of caffeine (100 mg or more) to generate a minor impact. Concentrated caffeine in this amount can increase anxiety, stress, and blood pressure.
- A dietary supplement from kidney bean extracts (known as Phaseolus vulgaris) is touted as a carbohydrate blocker because it temporarily deactivates an enzyme in the gut (amylase). Therefore, certain carbs cannot be completely digested and absorbed. The supplement seems to be able to deactivate the enzyme partially if taken before starchy meals (such as those with bread, pasta, or pizza). While there has been some minor weight loss reported, this supplement could also get you excited about eating more carbs and thus cause you to gain weight.
- Hydroxycitric acid (HCA) is a compound found in some tropical plants. It apparently blocks an enzyme that turns carbs into fat and may increase brain levels of serotonin, which acts as an antidepressant. Small amounts of weight were lost in a study that combined pill taking with walking. The dosage was generally 2 to 3 grams a day total, split before each meal and taken on an empty stomach. However, this pill in higher doses may also upset your stomach.
- Chromium is a mineral that potentially helps to regulate insulin or increase insulin sensitivity, especially in diabetics. Chromium may also help with metabolism. However, doses of 200 to 600 mcg (micrograms—very small amounts) have provided minor or no benefits in some studies.
- Conjugated linoleic acid (CLA) is a big seller, but there has always been a question of whether this product raises cholesterol (it is partially a trans fat) or C-reactive protein (an inflammatory marker), which are not desirable effects. It is a compound naturally found in meat and milk from cows,

goats, and sheep. It may prevent more fat from reaching fat cells. A one-year study found an average weight loss of 4 pounds. The usual dosage is about 3 grams per day, taking the pill with each meal. With the questions existing over cholesterol and other possible negative impacts and only a modest weight loss history in studies, this is probably one to avoid.

Prescriptions and Medical Procedures

Few prescription drugs are approved for long-term use with weight loss. These drugs come with catches, but they can help some patients who are desperately trying to lose weight and are willing to accept the potential side effects.

WEIGHT LOSS

Also known as cachexia, anorexia, and loss of appetite

What is it? Why does it happen? A substantial amount of weight can be lost during cancer treatment due to a loss of appetite, physical inactivity, and because of the effects of the cancer itself. Some cancers or tumors are responsible as they grow for the release of all kinds of compounds that cause the body to go into an accelerated metabolic state (hypercatabolic state). This condition should be addressed or treated because it can impact the quality and duration of a patient's life.

What are the signs or symptoms? Weight loss can occur throughout the entire body or in specific areas, and it involves not only the loss of muscle, but also of fat. At the same time, certain inflammatory compounds in the body, such as C-reactive protein (CRP) and fibrinogen, can be detected in increased amounts using blood tests. This is why some medications that reduce these specific blood markers are being tested to treat this problem.

Some HRPC clinical studies have referred to the phenomenon of weight loss as "anorexia," and in some ways the two are similar in that both are serious conditions, and the weight loss with each can be substantial. HRPC patients attempt to maintain their weight or gain weight, and to do so is very difficult in this situation. Identifying the underlying cause for the weight loss could allow for dramatic improvement. For example, if the weight loss is due to nausea or pain (with loss of appetite), depression, or fatigue, then aggressive measures should be taken to alleviate these symptoms. A two-pronged approach offers the best success—identify the cause with your doctor and work with a nutritionist who regularly helps cancer patients to come up with solutions for your situation.

Prevention and Treatment Options

Lifestyle and Diet Tips

- Even a minimal amount of daily exercise can increase or stimulate appetite, which will allow you to consume more calories. And, if your doctor gives you the okay then you need to also do resistance exercise (such as weightlifting) to increase your muscle mass, which will add some weight. Resistance exercise can be anything from lifting actual weights, to using large stretchable bands, to lifting canned goods several times a week. Health care professionals and trainers have come up with all sorts of ways to do resistance exercise outside of a gym if it is needed. When considering exercise if weight loss is a problem, you should avoid lengthy aerobic exercise that burns lots of calories. Stick with more moderate exercise until the problem is resolved.
- Consuming high-quality protein meals of beef, chicken, turkey, fish, and/or eggs can help to prevent muscle loss. For vegetarians, there are high-quality plant proteins such as soy and brown rice protein. The minimum goal is to get 0.8 grams of protein per kilogram (kg) of body weight (the recommended daily allowance), but recent studies are showing that 1.0 to 1.5 grams per kilogram can result in more improvement. Keep in mind that 1 kilogram of weight is equivalent to 2.2 pounds. A 200-pound person weighs about 91 kilograms; multiply that by 0.8 grams of protein, and you find that around 73 grams of protein should be the minimum daily target. Remember, a high-protein meal not only can help maintain muscle, but according to some recent studies it may also reduce the risk of nausea from chemotherapy.

- Dietary fat has the most calories per gram (compared to sugar and protein), which means that increasing your intake of healthy fats (monounsaturated and polyunsaturated) from nuts, seeds, and oils makes a lot of sense.
- High-calorie smoothie drinks or fruit drinks can contain tons of calories per serving and are also a good way to get more calories. High-calorie protein drinks from the grocery store are another option. Many companies, such as Abbott Labs, Nestlé, and others, make protein-based nutritional drinks and products for weight loss sufferers.
- Medical marijuana is now approved in several states in the United States. It is an option that should at least be discussed with your doctor because it does stimulate appetite. Tetrahydrocannabinol (THC) is one of the active ingredients in medical marijuana that are responsible for increasing appetite. This ingredient can also be found in a prescription drug that is used to increase appetite (see dronabinol, page 239). Of course, if you are considering this option, you would also need to consider the restrictions on operating machinery or driving a vehicle while using it.

Dietary Supplements and Over-the-Counter Options

Recently, combinations of dietary supplements and prescription medication approaches are becoming popular. The combined strategy seems to be more successful because each component treatment may target or block a different pathway in the body that is involved in weight loss. For example, a recent study combining fish oil and an anti-inflammatory prescription drug (such as Celebrex) appeared to be beneficial. Also, a recent phase-3 trial showed a benefit in combining a prescription progesterone drug (such as medroxyprogesterone [500 mg per day] or megesterol acetate [320 mg/day]) with EPA (fish oil, 2.2 grams), L-carnitine dietary supplements (4000 mg per day), and the drug thalidomide (200 mg per day). The combination worked better than any of these agents by themselves.

- One option mentioned in that study, L-carnitine dietary supplements, could be expensive, so compare prices. It was used in this clinical trial because blood levels of the compound have dropped significantly during extreme weight loss. There is no direct evidence as yet that L-carnitine by itself promotes weight gain, but it may help to improve energy levels during this time, which could be helpful. It is interesting to consider that the role of L-carnitine normally in the human body is to shuttle other compounds used for energy production in every cell.

- Fish oil dietary supplements taken in large amounts (2000 to 10,000 mg a day of the active ingredients EPA and DHA) seemed to promote weight gain in several studies. In fact, most of the data has centered on the EPA omega-3 fatty acid. Fats such as fish oil help promote weight loss when given in small amounts (1000 to 2000 mg/day), but in larger amounts they tend to cause the opposite effect, weight gain. It is interesting that, according to some studies, EPA or fish oil worked by maintaining muscle mass and not just by increasing the amount of fat in the body, which means combining it with a standard prescription medication such as megesterol acetate (Megace, see next page) makes more sense. Keep in mind that fish oil can also be a blood thinner in some individuals, especially those already taking other more potent blood thinners. Talk to your doctor before beginning use of this supplement.
- Dietary supplement protein powders that can be mixed with liquids include whey or egg white protein powder. They provide high-quality protein, and potentially can help reduce muscle loss. If you prefer a vegetarian protein option there are also soy and brown rice protein powders. It is important to get these supplements at least a total of 3 times a day following meals. In small amounts these supplements can suppress appetite, but in these larger quantities they could help to maintain muscle mass and provide a large source of calories. The amino acid leucine in the powders appears to be one of the most important stimulators of building muscle protein and possibly also maintaining muscle. Studies are currently underway with patients taking 500 to 1000 mg or more of leucine as a dietary supplement capsule in addition

to the leucine they are getting from the protein powders. It might be worth considering.

- Creatine dietary supplements also appear to be a safe way to add more protein and increase muscle building in individuals who are losing weight and still able to exercise. Creatine monohydrate supplementation appears to increase the energy capacity of the muscles during times of muscle loss and inactivity, which means it could improve workouts or at least help to maintain muscle. Several grams of creatine powder supplements can be used in addition to the protein powders.
- Vitamin D blood levels are usually very low in individuals who lose a lot of weight, and there is now some research to suggest that increasing your vitamin D intake to 1000 IU per day may help to stimulate muscle development. This makes sense, as there are vitamin D receptors on muscle tissue.
- Over-the-counter pain medications (also known as NSAIDs), such as ibuprofen, motrin, and naproxen, seem to reduce some of the inflammatory markers that increase with weight loss. If you are already taking these medications for pain, they may provide a 2-for-1 benefit in regards to weight loss.
- L-glutamine is an amino acid supplement that is an energy source for certain cells of the body, such as immune and gastrointestinal cells. It is recommended for some side effects from cancer treatment, but there is not much research regarding weight loss. If you need to use a dietary supplement in combination with a prescription drug, try using fish oil or L-carnitine. Both have at least been tested in large clinical trials and proven to be somewhat successful.

Prescriptions and Medical Procedures

- Progesterone drugs, primarily megesterol acetate (Megace, the most tested option) and possibly even medroxyprogesterone acetate (MPA), are some of the most effective treatments for weight loss. They increase body fat (not muscle) and stimulate appetite. In fact, in some countries, they are the only approved drugs for weight loss from cancer. These medications come in all different forms, including pills, liquids, and even injections. This option may increase the risk of blood clots when taken in high doses in rare situations. There is discussion as to whether this drug should be combined with other supplements and lifestyle changes.

- Steroids, such as prednisone or dexamethasone (Decadron), and others, can be taken as a pill and are already given to many men receiving treatment for HRPC. Steroids not only increase appetite, but also increase weight gain. Keep in mind that using higher doses of steroids is generally not an option for most patients because of concern about immune suppression with the increased dosage.
- Marinol (also known as dronabinol, delta-9-tetrahydro-cannabinol, delta-9-THC) can treat nausea, vomiting, loss of appetite, and weight loss. It is in a class of medications known as cannabinoids, which affect the same area of the brain as marijuana. It stimulates the area of the brain that controls appetite. When taken for appetite improvement, it is generally given as a capsule 2 times a day, before lunch and dinner, or it can be given in the evening. This may be a better option than smoking medical marijuana.
- There is also another prescription drug that is similar to dronabinol, known as nabilone (Cesamet). It is a pill that can be taken before and right after chemotherapy to reduce nausea and vomiting and also to stimulate appetite. These drugs have had limited success and may make the most sense in someone who is experiencing most of his weight loss due to nausea.
- Metoclopramide (Reglan, etc.) is a prokinetic agent, which means it speeds the movement of foods and beverages through the stomach. When given to some patients experiencing weight loss, it can improve the absorption of calories and nutrients. It may also work by allowing more food intake. It is a drug that can also reduce nausea, which may be another way it can help. It comes in a variety of forms—tablets, syrup, and injection. This drug does not generally facilitate the gain of significant amounts of weight, so it is not usually the first treatment choice.
- Prescription anti-inflammatory drugs, such as higher doses

of naproxen, ibuprofen, or even Celebrex (up to 400 mg per day), may help in combination with other products. Keep in mind that all of these pain-reducing medications have limitations based on your total health profile.

- There was a recent small study that used insulin treatment (the same insulin that diabetics use) to promote weight gain. Even beta-blocker drugs (blood and heart rate-lowering medications) may slow metabolism and possibly increase weight gain. Talk to your doctor about these options if others are not working.
- It may pay to look at HIV/AIDS research, since many drug clinical trials in this area study weight loss because it has been such a problem with advanced stages of the disease. For example, interest in the drug thalidomide came from HIV/AIDS studies in the 1990s. Thalidomide has promoted weight gain in some small studies of HIV patients and seems to be helping some cancer patients gain weight when used in combination with other products. An oral drug similar to thalidomide, known as Revlimid (lenalidomide), seems to also have the same weight gain–promoting properties.
- There is a non-steroidal selective androgen receptor modulator known as Ostarine. It is currently in clinical trials and appears to increase lean muscle mass, reduce fat, and perhaps increase energy levels. In addition, ghrelin is a hormone produced by the stomach and other areas of the body that increases appetite and food intake and also acts as an anti-inflammatory compound. Theoretically, if there were a way to increase the level of this hormone in the body, it could reduce weight loss. A synthetic form of ghrelin is being tested in clinical trials right now. Ask your doctor whether any of these newer treatments are available for use, and what are the benefits and risks.
- Growth hormone and testosterone are in general a big problem for patients with HRPC because there is a concern that they may promote tumor growth. This is true for most hormone therapies promoted to increase muscle mass and weight. However, if the weight loss is an extreme problem,

and nothing is solving it, then it may be time to consider a short course of these muscle-promoting hormones. Oxandrolone is a synthetic anabolic steroid derived from dihydrotestosterone (DHT). It works like other anabolic steroids and dramatically increases the amount of protein manufactured by the body to build muscle and increase body weight. This medication generally comes as a tablet that is taken several times a day.

- Please remember that if it is difficult for you to eat or drink for any time period, there are other nutritional options. Sometimes, "parenteral nutrition" is used that delivers a formula containing salts, glucose, amino acids, lipids, and added vitamins intravenously (IV).

A final thought to conclude the chapter on side effects: hopefully you've noticed that there are a multitude of treatments of every type to help prevent or alleviate the negative effects of cancer treatment. By utilizing some of the suggestions here, you can both improve the quality of your life during treatment and increase your chance of being able to continue the treatment successfully. Rather than suffering in silence, be sure to discuss any side effects you are experiencing or concerned about with your doctor to determine the best course of action in your individual situation. Knowledge is definitely power when it comes to side effects!

Diet, Supplements, *and* Alternative Medicine

Chapter Ten

Thus far we've discussed numerous treatment options for HRPC and methods of dealing with the side effects of those treatments. It is also worth considering some general tips to improve wellness while undergoing treatment, or in many cases, improving wellness overall.

Top Ten Dietary and Lifestyle Recommendations

Tip 1 If you are overweight or concerned about weight gain, a slight reduction in total calories from any food or beverage source is the goal. Keep in mind that reducing just 100 to 200 calories every day can help you to lose weight or maintain your weight. It does not matter where the reduction in the calories occurs—from juices, sugary sodas, half a candy bar, less rice, pasta, or bread … you pick!

Tip 1, Part II If you are underweight or trying to gain weight, a slight increase in total calories from any food or beverage source is the goal. Conversely, increasing your caloric intake daily by just 100 to 200 calories could help with weight gain. You can select the calorie source that you enjoy the most.

Tip 2 Breaking a sweat improves mental and physical health, but keep it moderate or it can make things worse. Getting a minimum of 30 minutes a day of movement time is a great tool to improve mental as well as physical health. However, during cancer treatment try to limit extensive or intense aerobic workouts to not more than every other day as opposed to daily because that activity level can actually increase fatigue. Your body takes longer to recover from a workout when there is less testosterone in your system and during cancer treatment in general, so exercising every day can actually make you more tired. You should work with your doctor to determine how vigorous your exercise program should be.

In general though, someone who is fit can calculate their maximum desirable heart rate by taking the number 220 and subtracting your age (for example, 220-50 = 170). Now, take that number and multiply by 0.50 (170 x 0.5 = 85) and 0.85 (170 x 0.85 = 145). In general, for this individual example, a good workout allows a minimum heart rate of 85 beats per minute and a maximum heart rate of 145 beats per minute. Be sure to check with your doctor to see how best to incorporate movement into your routine.

Tip 3 Weightlifting or resistance exercise just twice a week has diverse mental and physical health benefits. Ask your doctor if you can do upper and/or lower body weightlifting 2 or 3 times a week for 15 to 30 minutes each time. If it is possible, this can stimulate muscle growth, increase your metabolism, burn belly fat, reduce fatigue, reduce the risk of bone loss, and improve mental health during cancer treatment. If you are not allowed to lift weights because of your bone metastasis, try to do some light resistance exercise by doing swimming pool aerobics, walking, doing tai chi, or any other exercise that requires some movement and a little pressure on the muscles and bones.

Tip 4 Keep your cardiovascular disease risk to as close to zero as possible. Most heart-healthy changes have an anti–prostate cancer effect. It is a fact that too many men with HRPC die every year from heart disease, the number one overall cause of death in men. Therefore, considering heart health makes sense for everyone, including HRPC patients. LDL ("bad cholesterol") should be below 100 minimally, HDL ("good cholesterol") as high above 40 as possible, and triglycerides less than 100. Try to monitor your hs-CRP level to keep it low, and your blood pressure should stay within a normal range. It is interesting that virtually everything found to be heart healthy (exercise, weight loss, low cholesterol, low blood pressure) has turned out to have some anti–prostate cancer impact. If that weren't enough, another reason to follow your heart-healthy numbers is that they provide some real proof that any lifestyle change you are making is providing a benefit. For example, changing your diet or exercise can lower cholesterol and blood pressure and provides evidence to you that the changes you are making are actually helping you.

Tip 5 Healthy fats (monounsaturated and polyunsaturated) are your friends! Consume healthy fats, such as monounsaturated and polyunsaturated (omega-3) fats, which come from healthy sources, such as fatty fish, lean meat, nuts, plant oils, and seeds. Minimize saturated fat intake, not because it is unhealthy, but because most foods and beverages with higher amounts of saturated fat simply contain an excess of calories. You can select nearly identical beverages and foods and simply choose the one lower in saturated fat. Think about milk for a second: almond, soy, and skim milk contain no saturated fat and deliver 80 calories or fewer for an 8-ounce serving, but 2 percent and whole milk contain almost twice as many calories in the same serving!

Tip 6 Consume 20 to 30 grams of fiber a day, but not from pills or commercialized powders. Insoluble fiber and small amounts of soluble fiber (the 2 types of fiber) come from bran cereal, chia seed, flaxseed, legumes and beans, and low-calorie fruits and vegetables. Fiber helps prevent acid reflux, constipation, weight gain, and it lowers blood pressure, cholesterol, and even PSA in some studies. However, do not rely on fiber pills and powders for the majority of your fiber intake because they are much more expensive than fiber from food, contain mostly soluble fiber that can upset your stomach, and require enormous intakes to reach your 20 to 30 grams a day requirement. Did you know that most commercial fiber pills require anywhere from 10 to 60 capsules a day to reach your recommended daily allowance? No kidding! As an alternative, try just one third of a cup of bran cereal with a little flaxseed and fruit to provide 20 grams of fiber. As an added bonus, it will cost you very little!

Tip 7 The more you process food, the less the nutritional value and the more the calories! Think of any food in its natural state, for example, an apple. An apple is low in calories and high in fiber, but eating applesauce or apple juice means you consume more calories and little or no fiber. Generally, fruit and some vegetable juices are high-calorie inadequate substitutes for the real thing. Whole-grain bread, or even simple wheat bread, has better nutritional and fiber value as compared to plain white bread. Grass-fed beef has less saturated fat, more healthy fats, and just as much protein as less nutritious grain-fed or frozen patties of beef. Plain yogurt is more nutritious and contains fewer calories as compared to flavored yogurt or yogurt-flavored drinks. In other words, whenever possible try to pick foods that have not been processed to reduce your calories and increase your nutritious health benefits.

Tip 8 Sodium from the saltshaker is not the problem. Salt or sodium in excess can raise blood pressure. The recommended intake of 2400 mg per day to lower blood pressure can readily be achieved by reducing sodium from processed foods (check labels and pick the food that is lower in sodium). In reality, salt from the saltshaker is only a minor contributor to the total. In fact, in one of the most famous studies in the world (DASH), reducing sodium intake to 1500 mg or less along with diet changes and exercise, provided results equivalent to most blood pressure medications. Using small amounts of sea salt and spices is a great way to get more flavor from your food without using excess salt.

Tip 9 The "sin foods" or beverages are not the issue, and they may actually be beneficial. Alcohol, chocolate, ice cream, coffee, meat ... oh my! These things must be bad for you! Not really! In excess they are not heart healthy, but in moderation they can make you feel better and serve as a wonderful reward for following healthy lifestyle changes most of the time. In other words, maintaining a sense of normalcy is critical to maintaining overall mental and physical health.

One diet that has documented success is the Mediterranean diet. Research suggests that it has numerous health benefits as compared to other diet programs. If you look over the list of foods included in the Mediterranean diet, you'll find a diversity of healthy foods and beverages. It also promotes "everything in moderation" and includes foods and beverages that are not necessarily healthy for you. It appears that consuming more foods in moderation leads to more success than consuming several things in excess. It is also interesting that the Mediterranean diet does not involve taking a lot of dietary supplements or any other pills to prevent health problems.

Also worth noting is that many cancer books in the past suggested that coffee and caffeine were bad for you, but now clinical research suggests that consuming some caffeine from beverages can not only improve liver function, but also reduce fatigue. It may also prevent other diseases, improve mental health, and improve muscle recovery after workouts. However, in megadoses or when caffeine is taken from a pill, the concentrated form can increase heart rate and blood pressure, and is not heart healthy.

Tip 10 Stress, depression, lack of sleep, and other mental health issues are bad for your physical health, too. Whatever it takes—this should be your motto when it comes to mental health. You have to make sure that your mental health is as much of a priority as your physical health, and you should do whatever is needed to get there. Stress can dramatically increase your level of certain hormones that could have a negative impact on some cancer treatments. Stress can cause the release of abnormally high amounts of inflammatory substances and other compounds that can suppress your immune system, cause heart-unhealthy changes, and make it difficult to sleep and relax. If depression, stress, or anxiety is an issue, please seek professional assistance, counseling, more social support—whatever else is needed.

Tip 1 Skip the adult multivitamin. Adult multivitamins have too many ingredients that you do not need and that cancer cells may utilize for growth. In fact, one of the largest studies ever published on men with prostate cancer taking multivitamins found that they were not helpful and may have actually been harmful when the patients were getting too many multivitamins. Basically, despite adult multivitamins being the largest-selling supplements, there is no evidence to suggest that they help men with HRPC. If you feel compelled to take a multivitamin, take a children's multivitamin because these are the only multivitamins that do not have excessive dosages of a variety of ingredients that can be also used by cancer cells. In fact, while it is not known whether you need a children's multivitamin at all, the dosages at least are lower and appear to be safer. Be sure to select one with low amounts of folic acid because this B vitamin in supplements is also a concern (see next recommendation).

Tip 1, Part II Skip folic acid and any other B-complex dietary supplements. Folic acid is a B vitamin needed for cell replication, and folic acid is actually a target of many successful drugs in medicine that try to stop cell growth. Only a small amount of folic acid (400 mcg per day) is needed daily to provide help for normal body repair mechanisms, and this amount is easily consumed in many foods and most breakfast cereals due to fortification requirements aimed at reducing birth defects. The downside of the fortification is that today many men and women are getting too much folic acid. Umetabolized folic acid (UMFA) has been found in large amounts in men and women, and this occurs only when individuals get too much folic acid that cannot be utilized by normal cells, suggesting overconsumption. Research is showing that this excess may either increase prostate cancer growth or have no impact, but there is no consistent research that is demonstrating any benefit of getting folic acid from supplements for men with HRPC. Best to avoid folic acid supplements unless research indicates differently at some future point.

It is also important to prevent overexposure to other B vitamins, such as B12, because none of them in excess has been found helpful for men with prostate cancer. As with folic acid, excessive amounts from B complex dietary supplements could encourage cancer cell growth. Again, if you want or need to take a multivitamin, take a children's multivitamin.

Tip 2 Take a calcium supplement with vitamin D. Bone loss is a real problem when dealing with HRPC. Whether you are taking a prescription drug for bone loss or not, consider taking 1000 to 1200 mg a day of calcium from a calcium supplement with vitamin D. Calcium carbonate or calcium phosphate dietary supplements are the easiest and least expensive supplements to take because you need to take only 2 pills a day. However, take each pill with a separate meal if you can because the body does not absorb a lot of calcium at any one time. Try to take your calcium supplement with meals to improve absorption and reduce side effects. If you have a history of kidney stones or constipation, switch to a calcium citrate calcium supplement because it does not increase the risk of these problems. Calcium citrate can be taken with or without food (absorption is the same), but this supplement will cost a little more money.

Your calcium supplement should have enough vitamin D in it so that you are getting approximately 1000 IU of vitamin D a day. Most good calcium supplements have 250 to 500 IU of vitamin D per tablet, so getting enough vitamin D from your calcium supplement should be easy without taking too many pills. Never take more vitamin D than 1000 IU a day unless a vitamin D blood test suggests that you need more. A normal vitamin D blood level is 30 to 40 ng/ml (75 to 100 nmol/L).

Tip 3 Consider taking a fish oil supplement. Fish oil dietary supplements are not expensive and there are many reasons why they make more sense than most other dietary supplements for men with HRPC. Fish oil dietary supplements have been shown to potentially improve mental health (they reduce depression), reduce hot flashes, maintain normal blood glucose levels, lower triglycerides, increase HDL, lower blood pressure, reduce inflammation and arthritic joint pain, and perhaps help with weight issues. All of these benefits are exactly the main risks for men with HRPC, especially while their testosterone level is kept at the castrate level. The American Heart Association (AHA) recommends 1000 mg of fish oil a day for individuals with heart disease, but it would also make sense to recommend this same amount to most men with HRPC. The largest study of individuals without heart disease taking fish oil suggests that doses between 1000 and 2000 mg a day are more than enough. Be sure to discuss this supplement with your doctor, as it does have a blood thinning side effect that should be considered. Your doctor can help determine what dosage, if any, might be appropriate for your situation.

Tip 4 Consider taking a cholesterol-lowering drug (statin). While this is not a dietary supplement, if your LDL is greater than 100 mg/dL then you should discuss this possibility with your doctor. There is ongoing evidence to suggest that carrying abnormally high levels of cholesterol can encourage tumor growth. Whether or not that is substantiated through clinical studies, statins are one of the only preventive pills that can reduce the risk of the number-one cause of death in men and women—heart disease. Price should not be a concern, as many of the generic brands now cost almost what dietary supplements do. In addition, combining a cholesterol drug with fish oil has been found to provide a large benefit in one of the largest clinical trials to date, so the combination appears safe and beneficial for the individuals who need it. Discuss this one with your doctor. Remember, there are lots of ways to prevent or minimize statin side effects, such as decreasing the dose or frequency, changing the drug itself, or even taking creatine powder or Co-Q10 supplements.

Tip 5 Use protein powders to boost your protein intake. One of the most under-recognized problems in HRPC must be muscle or strength loss that occurs due to a low testosterone level (see the muscle loss side effect section in chapter nine). Lifting weights is one way to combat this problem, but new research also suggests that getting high-quality protein from lean meats, fish, and eggs may also help. However, it is not always easy to eat larger amounts of these types of proteins daily.

To supplement natural proteins, flavored whey or egg white protein powder can be very tasty when mixed with water, a sports drink, or your favorite beverage. It contains only about 100 calories, with approximately 20 grams of high-quality protein per serving! Clinical research suggests that consuming a protein powder daily can help to maintain muscle and strength, encourage weight loss or even weight maintenance, reduce nausea, and simply promote general health. Vegetarians can choose soy protein powder or brown rice powder, which are also good sources of non-animal-derived protein. It simply makes more sense for men with HRPC to use an evidence-supported protein powder daily as compared to taking a high-dosage multivitamin.

Miscellaneous Other Health Advice

ADRENAL ANDROGEN dietary supplements, such as over-the-counter DHEA and other advertised male hormone supplements, are in many cases similar to adrenal androgens, and they can still stimulate tumor growth. This is the case with DHEA and DHEA-like products, so please stay away from them.

ANEMIA supplements, over-the-counter pills, and even foods (wheatgrass is promoted in some places for this) to reduce the low red blood cell count due to cancer treatment are worthless, in most cases. They cannot fix or prevent anemia in HRPC patients because the anemia from prostate cancer treatment is usually caused simply by a lack of testosterone.

ANTIOXIDANTS (all of them) can also be pro-oxidants in the wrong situation. What does this mean? Too much of an antioxidant can create free radicals that do damage as much as they can stop free radical damage; hence they have pro-oxidant action. This is why going with the lowest dosage of any pill and being more skeptical as to whether or not you need a pill at all is the best way to go.

ARTHRITIS DIETARY SUPPLEMENTS are underrated. Arthritis dietary supplements are heart or kidney healthy (or at least not detrimental to your heart health) as compared to most prescription pain relievers for arthritis. So, fish oil, glucosamine, chondroitin, SAM-e, MSM, pycnogenol, and many other dietary supplements for arthritis seem to work better than a placebo, but more importantly they have an outstanding safety record (see the joint and muscle pain section).

ARTIFICIAL SWEETENERS are safe because they really do not get absorbed and do not change blood sugar levels. If you are using them to replace calories and sugar, then you will benefit. Millions of dollars have been spent studying these sweeteners (sucralose, aspartame, etc.) and research after 30 years continues to show they are safe. A natural sweetener, Stevia often gets lumped in as an artificial sweetener (see page 258 under natural sweeteners).

ASPARAGUS DIETS and other excessive vegetable-based diets are all over the Internet as a way to cure cancer. However, while there is no evidence to suggest that you can cure cancer with such a regimen, at least they appear to be safe. In the case of asparagus, it may cause your urine to smell strange because of the large number of sulfur compounds found in this vegetable. As long as a dietary change is heart healthy, feel free to try it. Considering such a diet instead of using a recognized cancer treatment is a problem because it can waste valuable time. However, changing to this diet or others along with receiving conventional treatment does not seem to be harmful and could be helpful in some cases.

ASPIRIN has anti-cancer effects. However, aspirin increases the risk of ulcers and potentially dangerous and deadly internal bleeding. Do not take aspirin daily for preventing any condition unless the benefits clearly outweigh the risks for you. Work with your doctor to accurately assess those benefits and risks.

BETA HCG injections, drops, or liquids for weight loss are a waste of money. Most programs include a radical reduction in total daily calories (fewer than 500 to 1000 calories a day!) along with the injections. Without the dramatic reduction in calories, would there be any benefit? The bottom line is that numerous clinical trials over decades have shown that this compound (beta-HCG) does not appear to increase weight loss, and it can cost you a ton of money to figure that out through your own "research."

CHELATION THERAPY While certain types of chelation therapy are used in traditional medicine, they are not the kind of chelation therapy used in alternative medicine for the treatment of cancer. Some people falsely promote chelation therapy as a way to reduce all sorts of toxins in the body and to help kill cancer cells, but this has never been proven or studied. Chelation therapy itself can be toxic to some of the organs and tissues of the body. Therefore, it is not recommended for the treatment of cancer.

COLON CLEANSING is not healthy because it involves having someone put a device in your bottom area (the politically correct term) and irrigate it with fluids. This can increase your risk of a serious infection, and the process is expensive. However, natural colon cleansing with fiber is brilliant! By consuming dietary fiber, such as All-Bran or another cereal daily, you can improve regularity, cleaning the entire area of the intestines that needs cleaning, and allowing more healthy bacteria to occupy your body.

CO-Q10 (also known as ubiquinone) is an expensive supplement that is primarily being tested in high doses to determine whether it helps slow the progression of Parkinson's disease. It is backed by minimal research to suggest it may reduce the side effects of statins (cholesterol-lowering medications) or lower blood pressure. However, it really has shown no benefit in prostate cancer thus far.

DRUG INTERACTIONS Every single time you start a new drug or over-the-counter pill, please research whether or ask if there are any interactions that can occur. For example, ketoconazole is a secondary hormonal drug that causes all sorts of drug interactions, and many substances also change the metabolism of the drug itself, such as grapefruit juice. Be sure to check to see if any foods, beverages, or other drugs interact with the treatment you are considering.

EGGS are a great source of high-quality protein, vision-improving compounds (lutein and zeaxanthin), and a source of vitamin D. They are low in overall calories, and the cholesterol should not be a concern for people who consume moderate amounts (1 or 2 eggs several times a week). They may be a good choice to boost protein intake.

ESSIAC TEA is made by combining 4 herbs—burdock root, Indian rhubarb, sheep sorrel, and inner bark of slippery elm. It was developed by a nurse in the 1920s and touted to treat breast cancer. Years later, an additional 4 herbs were added (blessed thistle, kelp, red clover, watercress) and that tea was also promoted to help all sorts of ailments. There is no real evidence that either tea fights cancer. However, it is possible that since it contains red clover, an estrogenic herb, some men with early stage prostate cancer may see a slight reduction in testosterone or PSA if using a large quantity, but there is a chance that those large amounts could also cause some liver toxicity. Overall, there are no studies to demonstrate whether this tea works for HRPC patients.

EXOTIC JUICES, such as goji, acai, and mangosteen, get a lot of hype, but they are expensive and have not been studied in men with HRPC. Since they can also be a large source of calories, if you do try these juices, please consume only a few ounces a day to avoid contributing to weight gain.

GARLIC SUPPLEMENTS are a waste of money, but natural garlic will always be found to be healthy. Garlic supplements may minimally improve your cholesterol or not, depending on which study you review, but the amount by which they reduce it is minimal when compared to red yeast rice or statin drugs. Additionally, garlic supplements can thin your blood, and that may not be a desirable effect. No research supports their value in HRPC.

GROWTH HORMONE (human growth hormone or HGH) has been advertised to cure, treat, or prevent just about everything. It comes in pill form, which is really worthless because the moment it hits the stomach the compound is deactivated by stomach acid. Anti-aging clinics charge a lot of money for injections of growth hormone that are supposed to help you maintain your muscle mass and give you extra energy. However, there is a big problem with growth hormone given to a cancer patient. Growth hormone also stimulates the release of large amounts of insulin-like growth hormone (IGF), and some of the potentially effective cancer drugs being developed today work to block the ability of IGF to get to a cancer. The extra quantity of growth hormone from an injection can continue to stimulate tumor growth. HRPC patients should avoid growth hormone injections.

KOMBUCHA TEA Sales of this so called “tea” are doing well. This is a “live” tea, which is really made by fermenting sweetened tea with yeasts and bacteria. Some companies suggest all types of benefits, but the studies are not matching all these claims. There are also case reports of upset stomach, allergic reaction, and even more serious immune problems so it is best to avoid this product.

LOW OXYGEN LEVELS Also known as "hypoxia." Basic scientific studies suggest that tumors with a low oxygen level may have a higher chance of recurrence or of being more aggressive. The theory is that when little oxygen is provided to a tumor it learns how to survive without an oxygen supply and becomes more aggressive in the process. There are some alternative medical clinics that promote oxygen therapy, but inhaling oxygen is not the same as providing oxygen at a microscopic level. In other words, you may be getting more pure oxygen, but this just gets utilized by larger organs and tissues and has never been proven to reach a tumor site. Also, inhaling pure oxygen from a tank, especially when it is not really needed, has the possibility of creating free radicals that could theoretically create more cellular damage.

LYCOPENE supplements have never lived up to the hype and should not be purchased. Foods, such as tomatoes or watermelon, are the best place to get dietary lycopene.

MACROBIOTIC DIET This is a specific food-type low-calorie diet that had some preliminary research long ago showing that it may help some prostate cancer patients. The majority of the diet (50 to 60 percent) is from whole grains, 25 to 30 percent from vegetables, 10 percent from beans (with a large focus on varied soy products), and several bowls of soup per day. On average, it seems that this diet really focuses on unprocessed or whole foods, and the average caloric count per day runs 1500 to 1800 calories at most. As a low-calorie diet, it can possibly help some people lose weight. The diet also encourages avoiding meat, eggs, dairy, and certain fruits based on an older philosophy, which does not necessarily reflect current scientific beliefs. Overall it is a healthy diet that does not encourage dietary supplements, but, it is not easy to get adequate intakes of vitamin B12 or vitamin D while following it. You would need to take certain nutritional supplements with this diet plan. Generally, any diet that is low in calories, healthy, but moderate in its approach is equally effective at being heart healthy and potentially having an anti-cancer impact.

MELATONIN This supplement helps individuals fall asleep, and it is also being tested for its ability to prevent neuropathy from chemotherapy drugs such as Taxotere. However, dosages of 10 to 20 mg have been given when only 0.5 to 1 mg is generally recommended for sleep. If you consult with your doctor and decide to try this for sleep and neuropathy reduction, start with the lowest dose to avoid taking more than you need.

MERCURY In general, smaller or tiny fish have less mercury as compared to larger fish because the older and larger the fish, the greater the potential for higher levels of mercury to accumulate in their bodies. For this reason, sardines, anchovies, and mackerel are used to make commercial fish oil pills that contain little or no mercury in them. King mackerel, shark, swordfish, and tilefish are large fish that can contain large amounts of mercury. Good commercially available fish to consume are:

Catfish (farmed)
Cod
Crab
Flounder or sole
Haddock
Herring
Ocean perch
Rainbow trout
Salmon (farmed and wild)
Sardines
Shellfish (crab, lobster, oysters, scallops, shrimp)
Tilapia (farmed)
Trout (farmed)

MODIFIED CITRUS PECTIN may help reduce PSA in some men because the product is loaded with fiber. However, there are cheaper sources of fiber, such as bran cereals, flaxseed, chia seed, veggies, beans, and whole wheat or whole grain products.

MUSHROOM immune boosting dietary supplements, such as Reishi and others, have been tested in a few clinical trials with no evidence of any benefit. These studies were small, but the promise of immune boosting and a clinical benefit has not been seen in patients with prostate cancer thus far. Companies boast about "beta-glucans" and other compounds found in these supplements that have demonstrated an impact in laboratory studies on immune parameters, but these have not translated into real clinical benefits. In fact, any supplement that claims an "immune boost" should potentially be avoided by HRPC patients because it could interfere with current drug treatments.

NATURAL SWEETENERS are not a bad idea. If something is sweeter than sugar, general research suggests you will use less of it. Stevia is 200 to 300 times sweeter than sugar, has no calories, and comes from a naturally sweet plant found in South America. It is sold in the U.S. in granular or liquid form. It does not cause your blood insulin or sugar to increase, and it tastes wonderful. Another sweetener, Sucant, has the same sweetness and calories as sugar, but it is unrefined, so it has more nutrients than sugar. Both agave and honey have slightly more calories than sugar but are sweeter, so you may be able to use less. You may want to consider trying some of these choices.

ORGANIC fruits, vegetables, and other products have not been proven to be healthier than less expensive (in most cases) non-organic fruits and vegetables. However, using less fertilizer and pesticide on foods not only is better for the environment but also, in some cases, may improve taste. For example, organic beef from cattle that were raised on grass tend to taste better. Economics can be your guide in this area.

pH BALANCED DIET The problem with these pH balanced products, such as specialty water, is that they somehow suggest that you can change the body's acidity or basic nature. This is really not possible. The theory is that cancer cannot survive in a basic environment, but it does well in an acidic environment. However, everything that hits the stomach gets bathed in an acidic environment, then is shuttled to the small intestine, where it becomes slightly basic in pH, and eventually is absorbed into the blood. The true problem is that the body controls the pH of the blood so strictly that even a tiny change would result in a medical emergency.

PROBIOTIC DIETARY SUPPLEMENTS These are a problem if you have advanced cancer because "friendly bacteria" are being taken by individuals who may have reduced function in their immune systems. While it is fine to get probiotics in foods, such as yogurt, it is a good idea to stay away from the supplements.

PYGEUM AFRICANUM This is a supplement for prostate enlargement patients that may improve urinary flow at a dosage of 100 to 200 mg per day. It has not been tested against prostate cancer. However, current prescription drugs for benign prostate hyperplasia (BPH) work very well and may have an added anti-cancer effect (dutasteride and finasteride), making them perhaps a better choice.

RED YEAST RICE EXTRACT No supplement is backed by more data and is more effective than a prescription statin (cholesterol-lowering) drug to reduce levels of bad cholesterol. However, if you are one of the few individuals who cannot tolerate a statin drug, then there are other prescription drugs out there that can help. If you cannot tolerate any cholesterol-lowering drug, then you can discuss with your doctor some potential supplements that may reduce your cholesterol, such as red-yeast rice extract. Still, you should be monitored by the doctor in the same way as if you were taking a prescription statin drug, because in reality you are taking a natural statin with red yeast rice extract.

RESVERATROL is more available as free reseveratrol in the blood when drinking red wine than taking most dietary supplements. Therefore, drinking red wine in moderation makes more sense than taking over-hyped dietary supplements of resveratrol.

SATURATED FAT from some sources is healthy. For example, getting a little saturated fat from nuts, seeds, plant oils, fish, and lean meats is healthy and can increase your good cholesterol. However, getting saturated fat from fast foods or high-fat dairy products gives you loads of calories that have very little nutritional benefit.

SAW PALMETTO is an interesting option for the treatment of prostate enlargement (BPH), but a few things need to be kept in mind. Current drug therapies for BPH work very well, and some may have anti-cancer effects (dutasteride and finasteride), so they may be better choices. Also, Permixon, a saw palmetto product tested in clinical trials that demonstrates efficacy, cannot currently be purchased in the U.S. Larger doses of saw palmetto (beyond 320 mg/day) may be more effective, but may also artificially reduce PSA levels in patients. There is no good data to suggest that these supplements have any impact on the risk of prostate cancer, but to improve urinary flow these supplements have helped a lot of men, and their safety record has been outstanding.

SELENIUM should *not* be taken as an individual supplement because it has been found to be unhealthy for the heart and skin in some studies because it increases the risk of type 2 diabetes or skin cancer recurrence. Getting selenium from a children's multivitamin or foods (fish, for example) is safer and should not make you feel worse.

SHARK CARTILAGE DIETARY SUPPLEMENTS have now gone through numerous clinical trials in cancer patients over the past 25 years, and *nothing* has been found that should lead anyone to take these pills. Additionally, they are difficult for the body even to absorb. Why contribute to reducing shark populations without research to support the product?

SOY Traditional soy products, such as soy milk, soy protein powder, tofu, tempeh, and soybeans, are low in calories, are high in protein, contain a good amount of fiber and omega-3 fatty acids, and should be consumed regularly.

SUGAR by itself is *not* backed by clinical research to show that it feeds cancer. Excess calories, excess weight, and excess insulin may feed cancer, and we know these changes increase your risk of cardiovascular disease. Calories and weight gain can come from excess carbohydrates (sugars), fats, or protein, and not just from sugar itself. As with many things, the key is to use sugar in moderation to feed your body's energy needs without contributing to weight or blood sugar problems.

TEA can be a good beverage if you enjoy a relaxing cup. While it contains a moderate amount of caffeine, it also has an anti-stress compound (L-theanine) and zero calories.

TRAVELING FOR ALTERNATIVE TREATMENT Some patients elect to travel to other countries for alternative treatments when they feel that they have run out of options. However, with off-label use of drugs, expanded access programs, clinical trials, and multiple physicians to consult, patients have ever-expanding options close to home. If you do choose to travel abroad for treatment, research the treatment, facility, and physician carefully to avoid possible serious complications.

URINE that is clear means that you are usually well-hydrated. When it is dark yellow, it generally means that you are dehydrated or getting B-vitamins from supplements. If it is another color, such as brown (liver or kidney), or murky and cloudy you should see your doctor.

VITAMIN C supplements have been found to be very safe even in doses of 500 to 1000 mg per day. However, vitamin C is very acidic; hence its other name "ascorbic acid."If you have a sensitive stomach, you should use a buffered vitamin C or calcium ascorbate. Megadoses of vitamin C supplements have not been effective in fighting cancer, but may have improved quality of life in some individuals who receive it in larger doses when their cancer is very advanced.

VITAMIN E supplements are a waste of money. They have been tested in many, many clinical trials and they have been found to be ineffective against heart disease or cancer. They may even reduce the efficacy of some cancer treatments.

WATER FILTER Most tap water across the U.S. is arguably some of the safest in the world. However, some advanced cancer patients have reached a point where their immune systems are very low or suppressed; they cannot afford to battle an infection, even if it is a small infection. If an individual is concerned about the water from a well or public source, here are some tips to consider:

- Have your water tested or get a copy of the consumer confidence report that most water utilities are required to send out by mail every July 1 or post on the utility web site. If there are increased levels of any contaminants in your water, find a water filter that has been certified to reduce these contaminants. You can purchase an activated carbon filter that is certified to reduce lead, cysts (from microorganisms), and volatile organic compounds (VOCs). Also, the filter should be certified to eliminate the impact of chlorine on the taste and smell of the water. Filtering out these items will provide simple, basic protection against disinfection byproducts, pesticides, and other chemicals.
- If you are concerned about bacteria and viruses, get a system or water filter that has been certified by an organization such as the Water Quality Association (WQA), NSF International, or Underwriters Laboratories (UL). The filter should have

pores so small it does not allow microorganisms to pass through, or it should use ultraviolet light to disinfect the water.

- The most costly option if you are really sensitive about the purity of your water: consider buying a reverse osmosis–and–activated carbon system. Finally, add a filter that has been certified for microbiological purity. This option is expensive, and it wastes several gallons of water for every gallon filtered. It can also filter out important minerals along with the contaminants, such as calcium and fluoride.

WATER-SOLUBLE VITAMINS SUPPLEMENTS can actually be dangerous! There is a belief that taking too much of a water-soluble vitamin is okay because the body will dump the excess in urine. However, other than giving you expensive urine, taking too much folic acid or other B vitamins could also potentially stimulate tumor growth. Just because a vitamin is water-soluble does *not* mean that it is safe in excess!

ZINC should not be taken in high doses. Just 11 mg a day for men and 8 mg a day for women is the recommended daily allowance. There is also some suggestion that getting more zinc from supplements may improve the taste changes that occur with some chemotherapy drugs (see the taste changes side effect section in chapter nine). Otherwise, getting more zinc than is found in a children's multivitamin for long periods of time is not worth it, again unless there is a specific reason for increasing your zinc intake.

ZERO = your heart disease risk. While practically it is impossible to reduce any risk to zero, you should pursue lifestyle changes and take supplements that have proven to be heart healthy because these are the ones most likely to have an anti–prostate cancer effects. Additionally, "zero" should represent your tolerance for taking any pill without completely analyzing whether the benefit outweighs the risk. Most HRPC patients should avoid taking any supplements unless there is a specific side effect or condition that requires it. Always consult with your doctor before adding any new supplement or over-the-counter medication to your treatment regime.

As we reach the end of this book, we hope that we've been successful in presenting you with a wealth of information on treatment options for HRPC and useful tips for managing your treatment side effects. The content here is meant to provide a basis for continuing discussions with your doctor to determine the best course of action for your individual situation. As noted, research continues all the time, and new treatment options regularly become available, so it always important to continue to expand your knowledge about the disease. Always remember, knowledge and action equal power in dealing with your cancer!

Notes

For additional information on improving diet.

Dr. Moyad's No Bogus Science Health Advice

A Step-by-Step Guide to What Works and What's Worthless.

ISBN: 978-1-58726-256-2

$19.95

Telephone 877-722-2264

www.info@aaeditions.com

Appendices

First appendix

OFF-LABEL DRUGS

The following drugs have been FDA approved for treatment of another cancer or condition. While they have not been studied or specifically approved for use in HRPC, they can be used "off label" if your doctor feels that they might be helpful. This is only a partial listing as the possibilities used by doctors change regularly with continuing research. Be sure to check with your doctor on these or other drugs that may help with your cancer.

Albumin-bound paclitaxel

Also known as Abraxane

How is it taken? IV

Company Celgene

Quick comment Drug blocks cell division and is really an advanced form of the chemotherapy drug Taxol®, which may provide better drug delivery for maximal efficacy and fewer side effects.

Bevacizumab

Also known as Avastin

How is it taken? IV

Company Genentech

Quick comment Angiogenesis-inhibitor drug that blocks a compound known as VEGF-A. A HRPC phase-3 clinical trial that used this drug in combination with Taxotere chemotherapy did not show a benefit greater than getting Taxotere alone, so the future of this drug in HRPC treatment is now uncertain.

Calcitriol or prescription vitamin D

Also known as Rocaltrol, Calcijex, and other names

How is it taken? pill

Company multiple companies

Quick comment A phase-3 trial using high doses of these medications with Taxotere chemotherapy for men with

HRPC did not show a benefit greater than getting Taxotere alone, so the future of this drug in HRPC is now uncertain.

Candesartan

Also known as Atacand and other names

How is it taken? pill

Company AstraZeneca and Takeda

Quick comment This is an angiotensin-2 receptor antagonist that has been preliminarily shown to block blood vessel growth and reduce PSA in some men with HRPC. The drug is already used to treat high blood pressure.

Capecitabine

Also known as Xeloda and others

How is it taken? pill

Company Genentech & Roche

Quick comment A chemotherapy drug that blocks DNA synthesis in the tumor. It is well known in breast and colon cancer treatment, used in combination with other chemotherapy drugs.

Celecoxib

Also known as Celebrex

How is it taken? pill

Company Pfizer

Quick comment This is a COX-2 inhibitor or pain-relieving drug that reduces inflammation. It has been shown to increase the risk of cardiovascular disease. It has been combined with multiple cancer drugs in smaller studies to determine whether it helps eliminate cancer cells.

Cholesterol-lowering drugs

Also known as statins

How is it taken? pill

Company multiple companies

Quick comment These drugs are some of the most popular in the world to prevent heart disease, and they are being studied in combination with other drugs to determine whether they enhance the tumor killing impact of some treatments.

Carboplatin

Also known as Paraplatin
How is it taken? IV
Company Bristol-Myers Squibb (Paraplatin) or Sanofi-Aventis
Quick comment This drug is known as an alkylating agent that interferes with DNA. It has been combined with other chemotherapies, such as Taxotere, in some smaller studies, and is somewhat similar to the drug oxaliplatin.

Cyclophosphamide

Also known as Cytoxan
How is it taken? pill
Company multiple companies
Quick comment Low doses of this drug seem to stimulate the immune system (higher doses depress the immune system). It may also prevent tumors from forming their own blood supply and it has a low rate of side effects.

Dasatinib

Also known as Sprycel
How is it taken? pill
Company Bristol-Myers Squibb
Quick comment This is an SRC inhibitor or multi-target tyrosine kinase inhibitor. It also has a phase-3 trial ongoing involving men with HRPC.

Doxorubicin

Also known as Adriamycin, Rubex, and other names
How is it taken? IV
Company Pharmacia, Upjohn, and Bristol-Myers Squibb
Quick comment Drug is known as an anthracycline that interferes with DNA and has been combined with other chemotherapy drugs in some smaller studies.

Epirubicin

Also known as Ellence
How is it taken? IV
Company Pfizer
Quick comment An anthracycline chemotherapy drug that is somewhat similar to doxorubicin; it interferes with

DNA. It has been combined with other chemotherapy drugs in other small studies.

Erlotinib

Also known as Tarceva

How is it taken? pill

Company Genentech and OSI

Quick comment EGFR tyrosine kinase inhibitor that is being tested in HRPC.

Everolimus

Also known as Afinitor

How is it taken? IV or pill

Company Novartis

Quick comment An mTOR inhibitor, which means it blocks the action of an abnormal protein inside the cancer cell that controls growth-related functions. It is used primarily now for advanced kidney cancer, which is why it is getting interest in other areas. It is somewhat similar to the drug temsirolimus.

Gemcitabine

Also known as Gemzar

How is it taken? IV

Company Eli Lilly

Quick comment A chemotherapy drug that blocks cancer cell growth.

GM-CSF

Also known as Leukine, Sargramostim, and others

How is it taken? injection

Company Genzyme

Quick comment These drugs are used primarily in HRPC to reduce the risk of several different side effects from chemotherapy, such as a low white blood cell count (neutropenia), which means the drug also has some immune-stimulating properties.

Ixabepilone

Also known as Ixempra

How is it taken? IV

Company Medarex, Inc. and Bristol-Myers Squibb

Quick comment Somewhat similar to the drug patupilone; is usually combined with other chemotherapy drugs.

Lenalidomide

Also known as Revlimid

How is it taken? pill

Company Celgene

Quick comment Known for its favorable impact on multiple myeloma, lenalidomide is being tested in a phase-3 trial of HRPC patients in combination with Taxotere chemotherapy.

Oxaliplatin

Also known as Eloxatin

How is it taken? IV

Company Bristol-Myers Squibb (Paraplatin) or Sanofi-Aventis

Quick comment This drug is known as an alkylating agent that interferes with DNA. It has been combined with other chemotherapies such as Taxotere in some smaller studies, and is somewhat similar to the drug carboplatin.

Sorafenib

Also known as Nexavar

How is it taken? pill

Company Bayer and Onyx

Quick comment Well known with kidney and other cancers as a way of blocking cancer blood vessel growth. This drug is somewhat similar to the drug sunitinib (Sutent®), which was not effective in a recent phase-3 clinical trial for men with HRPC.

Temsirolimus

Also known as Torisel

How is it taken? IV or pill

Company Pfizer

Quick comment An mTOR inhibitor, which means it blocks the action of an abnormal protein inside the cancer cell that controls growth-related functions. It is used primarily now for advanced kidney cancer, which is why it is getting interest in other areas.

It is somewhat similar to the drug everolimus.

Testosterone

Also known as Androgel, Testim, Testopel, and others

How is it taken? gel, injection, patch, pellet, pill

Company multiple companies

Quick comment Surprisingly, testosterone is being studied in some smaller studies of men with HRPC to determine whether some cancer cells are actually inhibited by testosterone, or may respond again to other hormone-sensitive cancer drugs when exposed to some testosterone again.

Thalidomide

Also known as Thalomid

How is it taken? pill

Company Celgene

Quick comment Known for its favorable impact on multiple myeloma, this drug is similar to the drug lenalidomide.

Vinblastine

Also known as Velban

How is it taken? IV

Company Pierre Fabre and multiple companies

Quick comment An anti-mitotic chemotherapy. It is usually combined with other chemotherapy drugs, and is somewhat similar to the drug vinorelbine.

Second appendix

PHASE 1 AND 2 CLINICAL TRIALS

Following is a listing of some of the drugs currently in phase 1 or 2 testing. Please note that research moves so quickly that these drugs may or may not be available, and more drugs get added and deleted to the list on a regular basis.

AT-101

Also known as R-(-)-Gossypol Acetic Acid
How is it taken? pill
Company Ascenta Therapeutics, Inc.

Cilengitide

Also known as EMD121974
How is it taken? IV
Company Merck Serono

Cixutumumab

Also known as IMC-A12
How is it taken? IV
Company ImClone Systems Inc.

Eribulin mesylate

Also known as E7389 or Halichondrin B analog
How is it taken? multiple delivery systems
Company multiple manufacturers

Figitumumab

Also known as CP-751,871
How is it taken? IV
Company Pfizer

Licochalcone-A

Also known as extract from Glycyrrhiza glabra (licorice root)
How is it taken? pill
Company To be determined

Patupilone

Also known as Epothilone B/EPO906
How is it taken? IV
Company Novartis Pharma AG

Pertuzumab

Also known as 2C4 or Omnitarg

How is it taken? IV

Company Genentech

Ridaforolimus (formerly known as Deforolimus)

Also known as MK-8669

How is it taken? pill

Company Merck and Ariad

Sagopilone

Also known as ZK-EPO

How is it taken? IV

Company Bayer

Sodium butyrate

Also known as Butyryl triglyceride

How is it taken? pill

Company multiple manufacturers

Tasquinimod

Also known as ABR-215050

How is it taken? pill

Company Active Biotech

TOK-001

How is it taken? pill

Company Tokai

Tributyrin

Also known as butyrate prodrug

How is it taken? pill

Company multiple manufacturers (moving to phase-3 trial now)

Vadimezan

Also known as ASA404

How is it taken? IV

Company Novartis & Antisoma

Vandetanib

Also known as Zactima

How is it taken? pill

Company AstraZeneca

Third appendix

IMAGING TESTS USED IN PROSTATE CANCER

A variety of imaging tests are used to give physicians a reliable analysis of the location and possible spread of your cancer. Many of these tests are used to provide a baseline when compared to the same test at a later date. For example, comparing a recent bone scan to a bone scan from months or years ago can help determine if bone metastasis or further spread of the cancer has occurred. These tests may lead to further tests or treatments, such as a biopsy, the removal of a lymph node, or the treatment of an area of the body to eliminate tumor cells. Most of these imaging procedures are painless, with the possible exception of a needle stick to inject dye to improve readability of results.

Bone Scan

Advantage A bone scan, also called a "radionuclide bone scan" or "bone scintigraphy," is the gold standard test for determining if a patient has prostate cancer that has spread to any of the bones.

The catch The test exposes the patient to radiation and may not be able to pick up very tiny bone metastasis. It can appear falsely positive for cancer if the patient has arthritis, degenerative bone disease, infection, or fracture.

Computed Tomography (CT scan)

Advantage A CT scan can find cancer in the regional and non-regional lymph nodes, especially when the nodes become large in size because the test detects this size change. It is a good complementary test to investigate a suspicious region found on bone scan or plain x-ray.

The catch The test exposes the patient to radiation and until the lymph node becomes larger in size it cannot detect a possible cancer in that location.

Intravenous Pyelogram (IVP)

Advantage An IVP is used to provide an image of the

kidneys, ureters, and bladder.

The catch The test exposes the patient to radiation. It is rarely used any more because newer devices are preferred.

Magnetic Resonance Imaging (MRI)

Advantage An MRI does not involve exposure to radiation. It may be able to find cancer in and around the prostate, such as the seminal vesicles or regional lymph nodes (stage N1). MRI can even find tumors in the spine, especially some high-grade tumors.

The catch MRI is not good at detecting cancer in the lymph nodes unless a special iron oxide dye is used. It is not as useful as a bone scan for finding cancer in bony areas. Because the test utilizes a strong magnet, it cannot be used on individuals with metal in their bodies, such as from past medical procedures.

PET/CT Scan

Advantage This technology is rapidly developing. It may be able to pick up cancer in the organs, bone, or non-regional and regional lymph node metastasis very early when the nodes are still not large enough to be picked up by CT scan or MRI. It can sometimes detect cancer when a bone scan did not find cancer in the bones because it relies on a tracer compound to find even tiny tumors.

The catch The patient is exposed to radiation. Finding the right tracer marker (carbon-11, choline, glucose, NaF) to be used with the test is challenging because the technology is developing so quickly. In some cases, patients have problems with insurance coverage for this test.

ProstaScint Scan

Advantage The ProstaScint scan can suggest whether or not cancer has returned after localized treatment for prostate cancer, especially in the areas around the prostate.

The catch This test is of little value for a man with HRPC.

Also, the accuracy of this test has been questioned.

Transrectal Ultrasonography (TRUS)

Advantage A TRUS involves no radiation exposure. It is the gold standard device to obtain prostate tissue biopsy samples.

The catch The TRUS is not a good test by itself for detecting a tumor in or near the prostate.

X-ray

Advantage In traditional x-ray procedures, the patient receives a low amount of radiation exposure. The tests can be done quickly.

The catch X-rays only show something when it is more obvious and takes up a lot of space, such as an infection, fracture, or cancer in the lungs or the ribs. They are not as good at finding small-to-moderate amounts of cancer or bone loss.

Fourth appendix

ADVOCACY AND SUPPORT ORGANIZATIONS

Alliance for Prostate Cancer Prevention www.apcap.org

American Cancer Society www.cancer.org

American Society of Clinical Oncology www.asco.org

American Urological Association www.auanet.org

CancerCare www.cancercare.org

Chemotherapy Care www.chemocare.com

Clinical Trials Recruiting, Ongoing & Completed www.clinicaltrials.gov

Foundation for Cancer Research and Education www.cancer-foundation.org

HRPCa.org. www.hrpca.org

MaleCare www.malecare.org

Man to Man, local groups of the American Cancer Society www.cancer.org

Malecare Advanced Prostate Cancer Program www.advancedprostatecancer.net

National Alliance of State Prostate Cancer Coalitions www.naspcc.org

National Comprehensive Cancer Network www.nccn.org

Patient Advocates for Advanced Cancer Treatments www.paactusa.org

Prostate Cancer Foundation www.pcf.org

Prostate Cancer Info Link http://prostatecancerinfolink.net

Prostate Cancer Research and Education Foundation www.pcref.org

Prostate Cancer Research Institute www.prostate-cancer.org

Prostate Conditions Education Council www.prostateconditions.org

Prostate Forum www.prostateforum.com

Prostate Health Education Network, Inc. (PHEN) www.prostatehealthed.org

The Prostate Net www.prostate.net

Us TOO International Prostate Cancer Education and Support Network www.ustoo.org

Zero—The Project to End Prostate Cancer www.zerocancer.org

Index

(illustrative material is shown in italics)

D

E

F

G